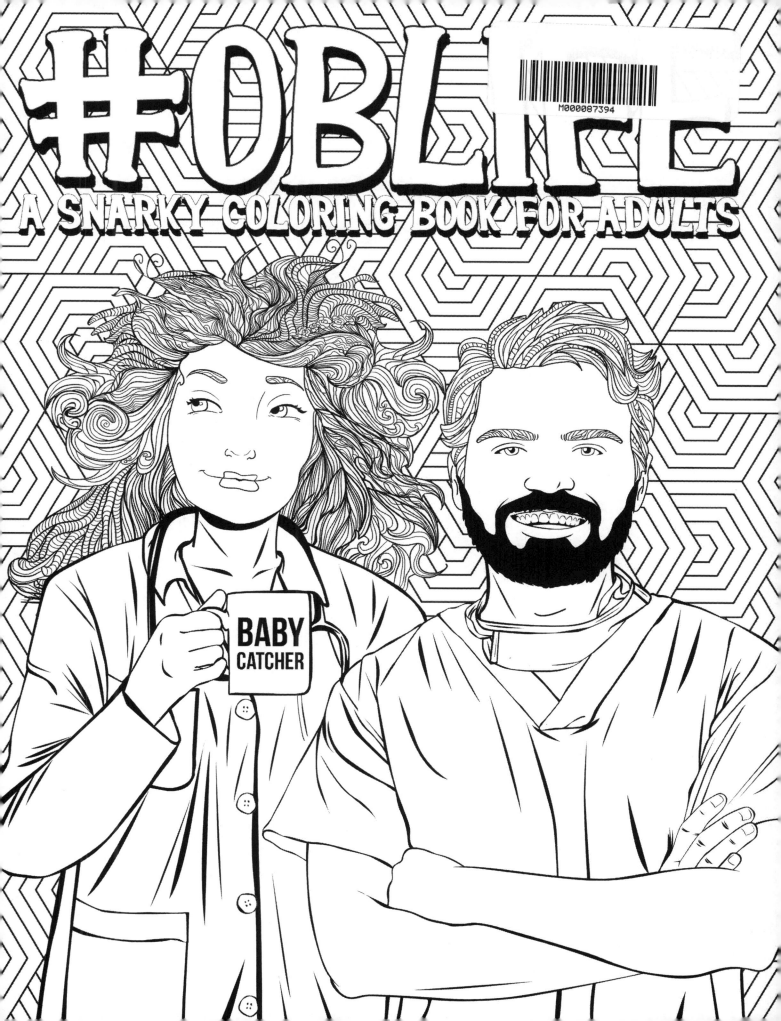

Want free goodies?
Email us at freebies@pbleu.com

@papeteriebleu

Papeterie Bleu

Shop our other books at
www.pbleu.com

Wholesale distribution through Ingram Content Group
www.ingramcontent.com/publishers/distribution/wholesale

For questions and customer service, email us at
support@pbleu.com

FREE PDF DOWNLOAD
OF THIS BOOK

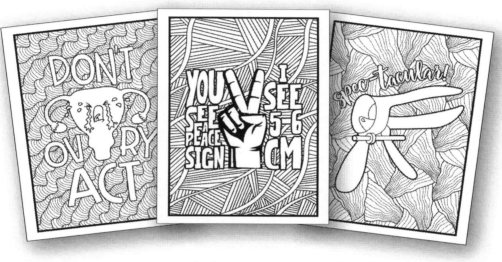

www.pbleu.com/baby

YOUR DOWNLOAD CODE: GYN373

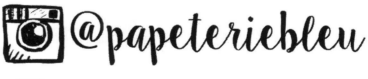 @papeteriebleu

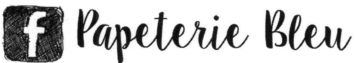 Papeterie Bleu

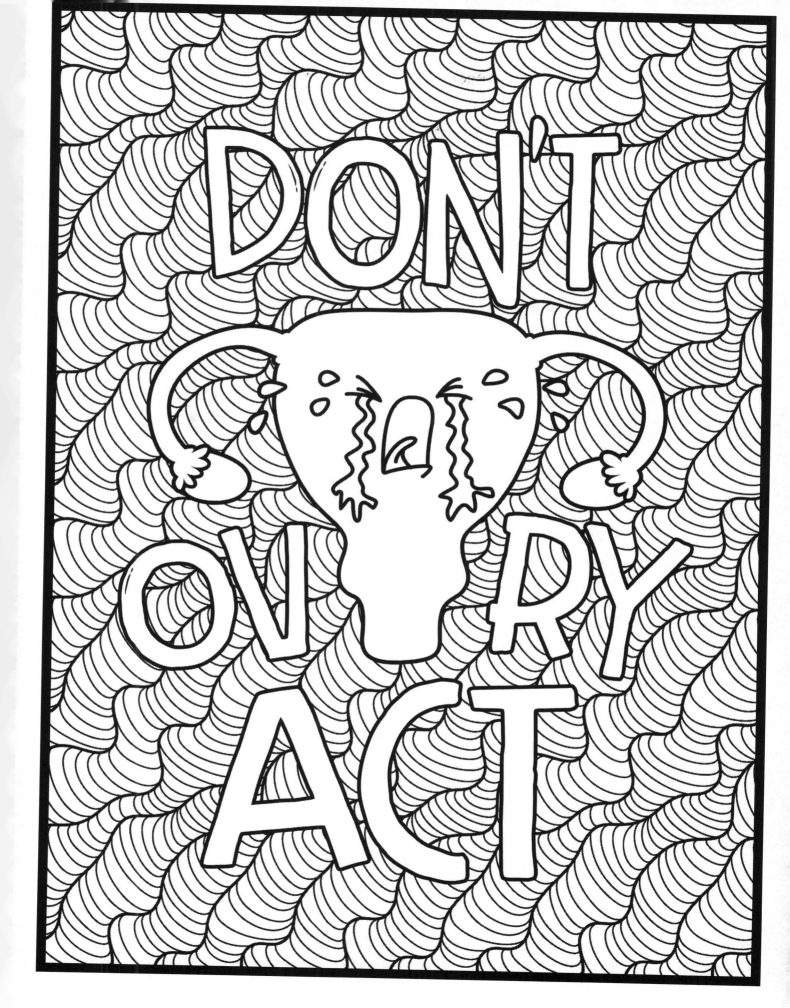

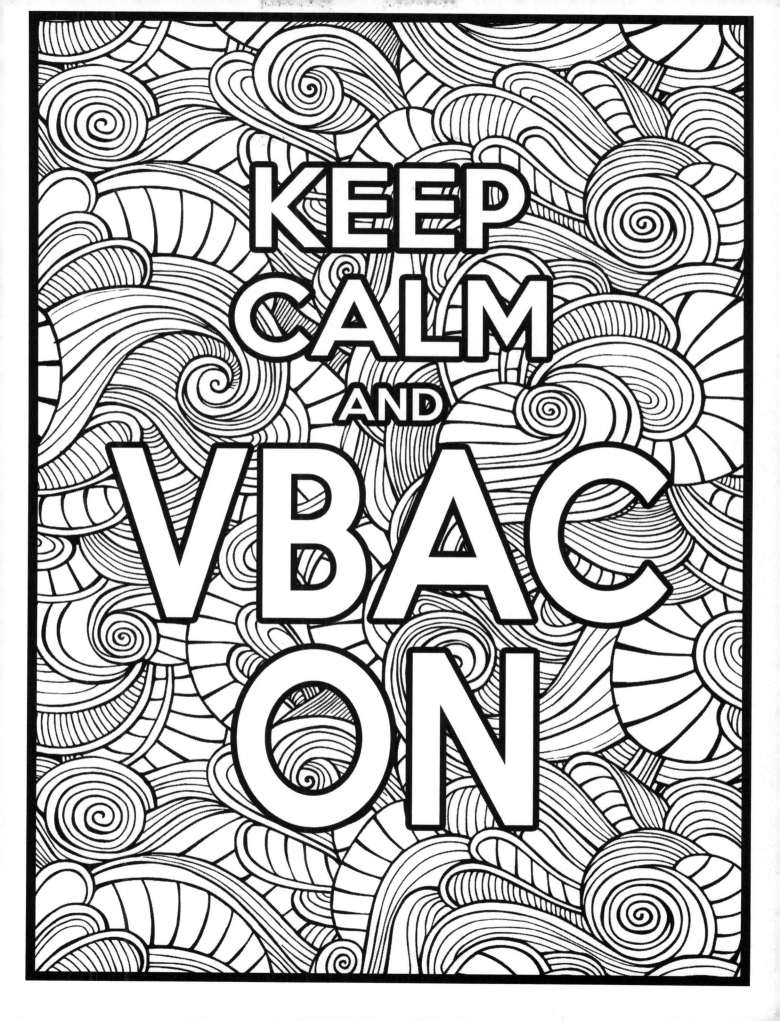

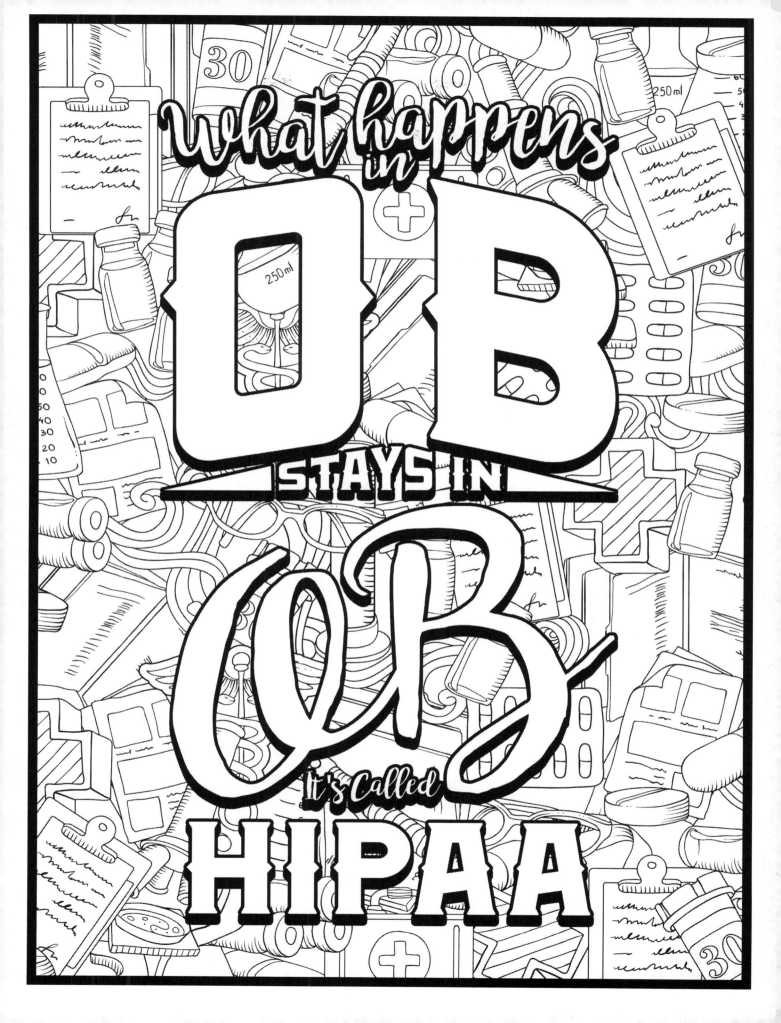

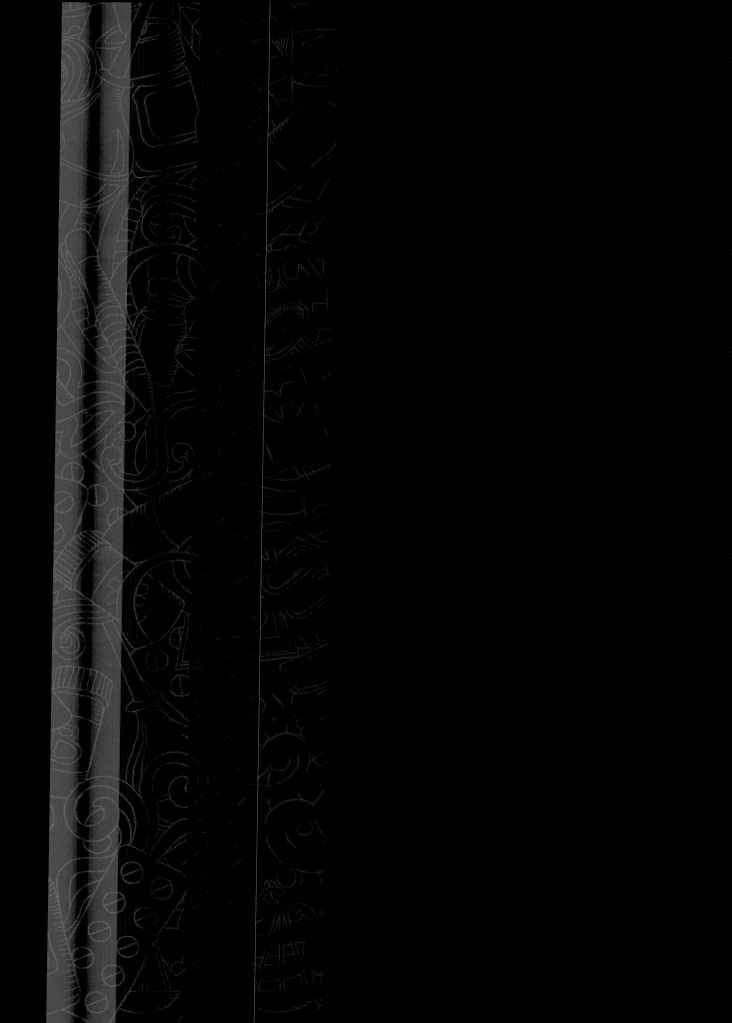

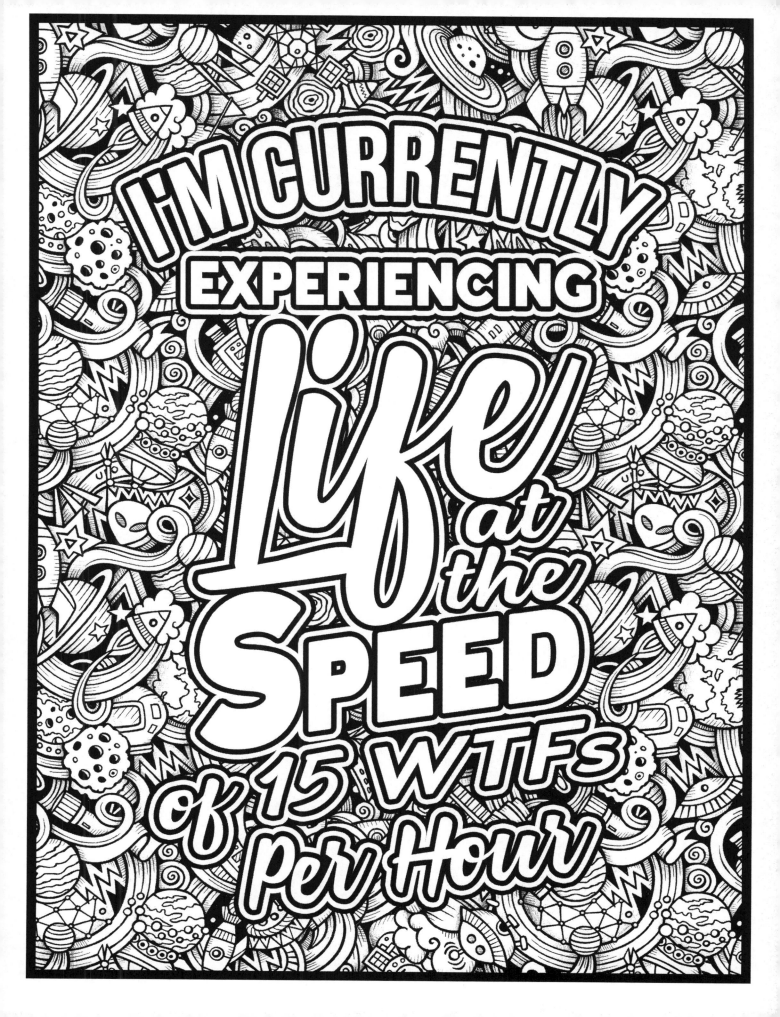

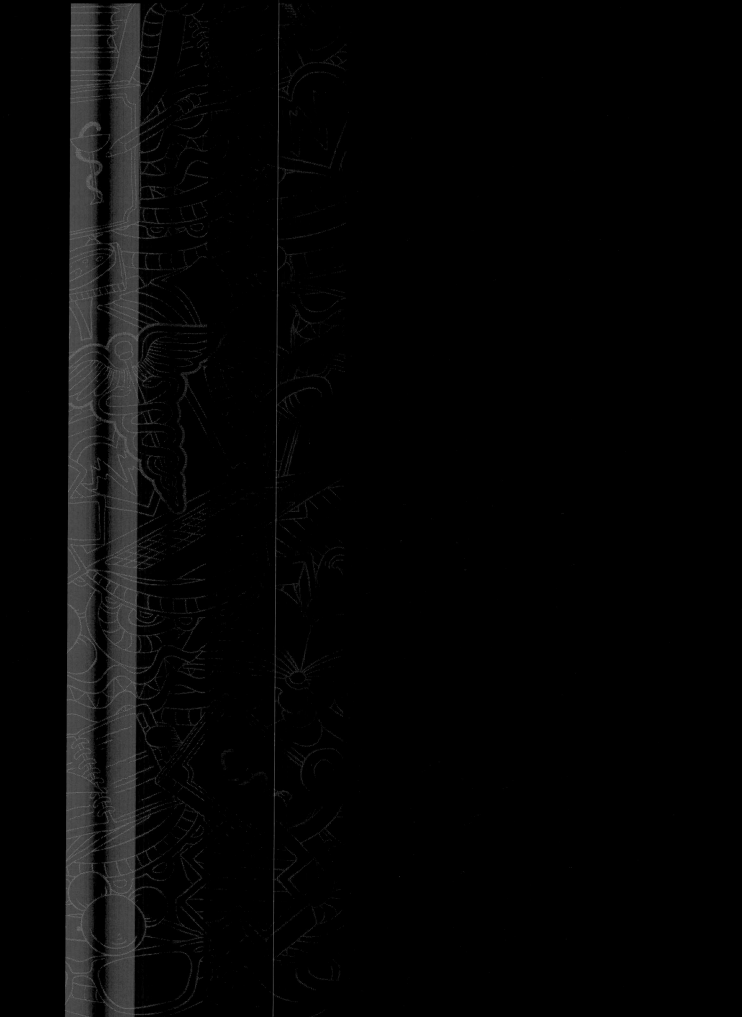

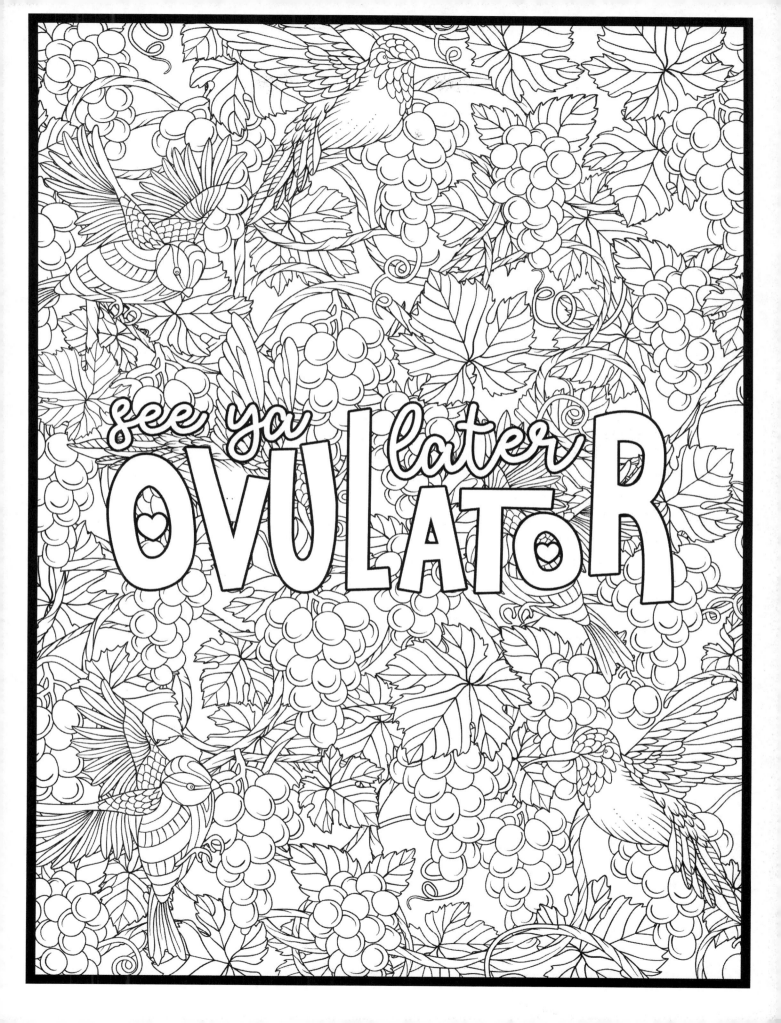

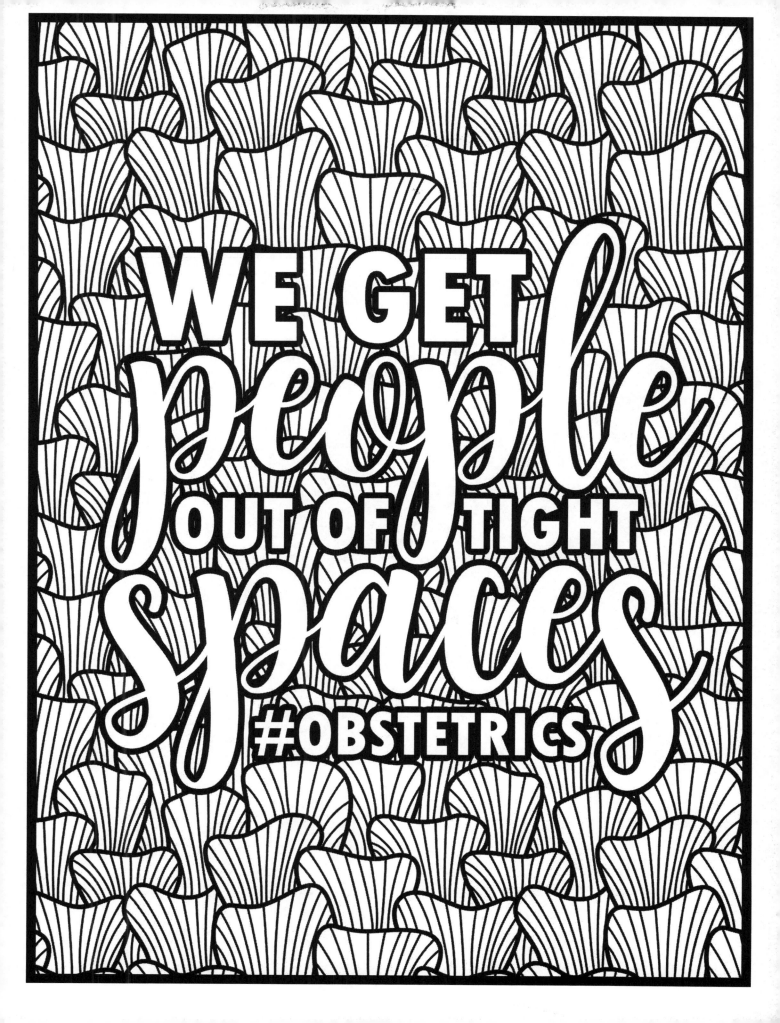

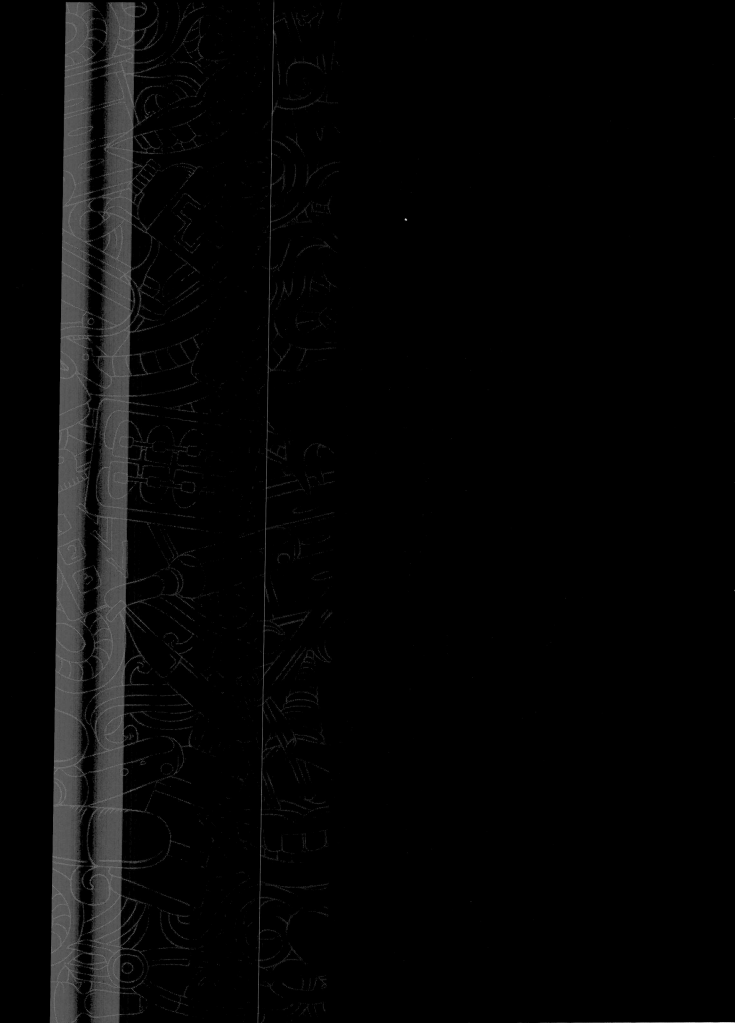

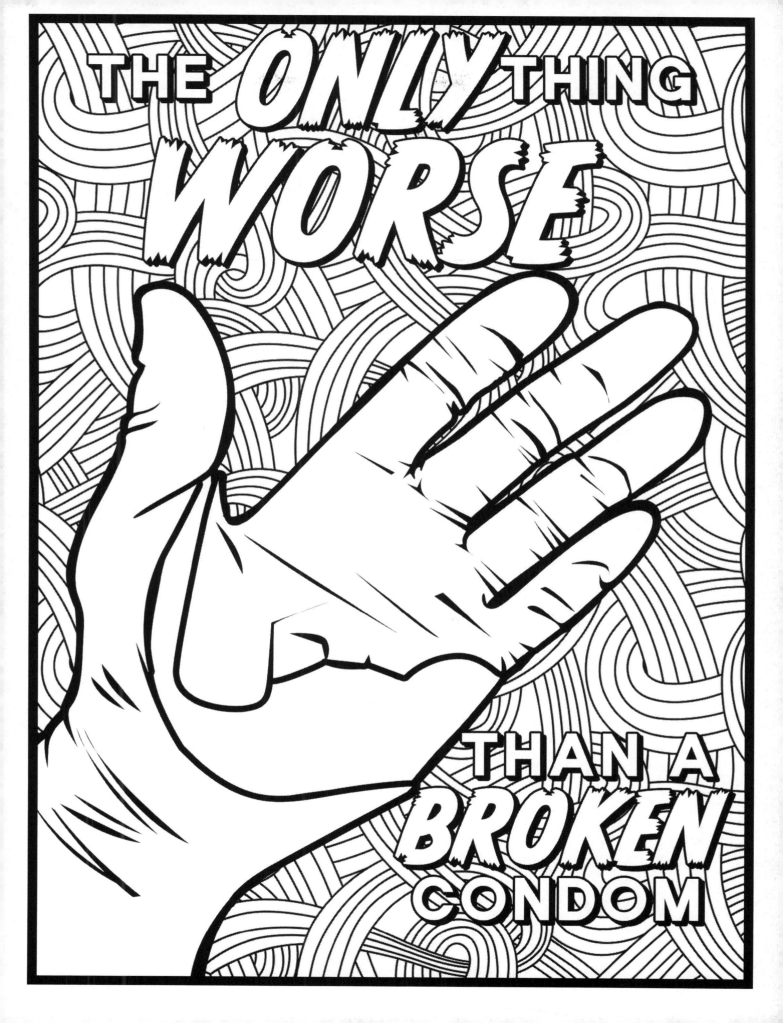

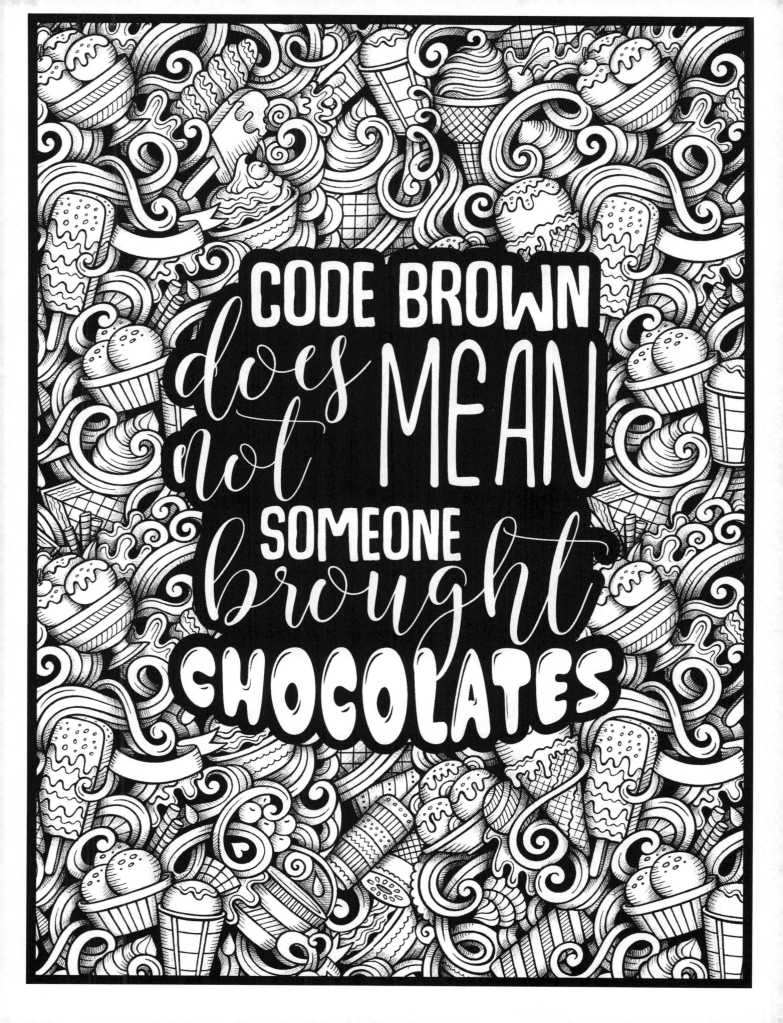

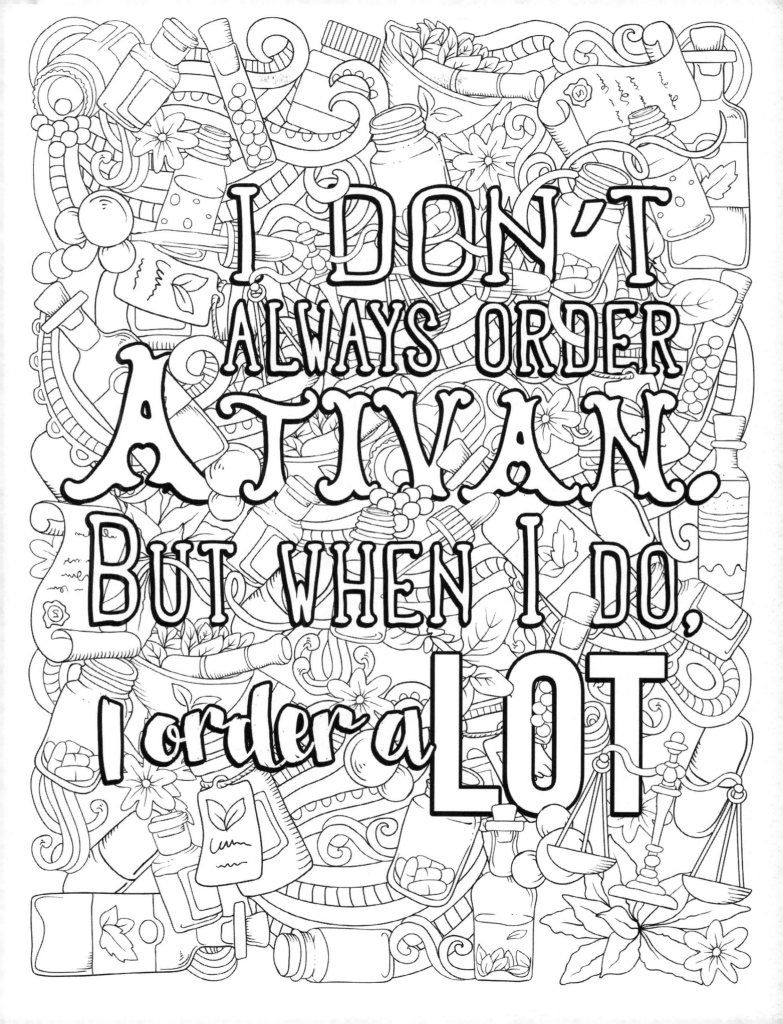

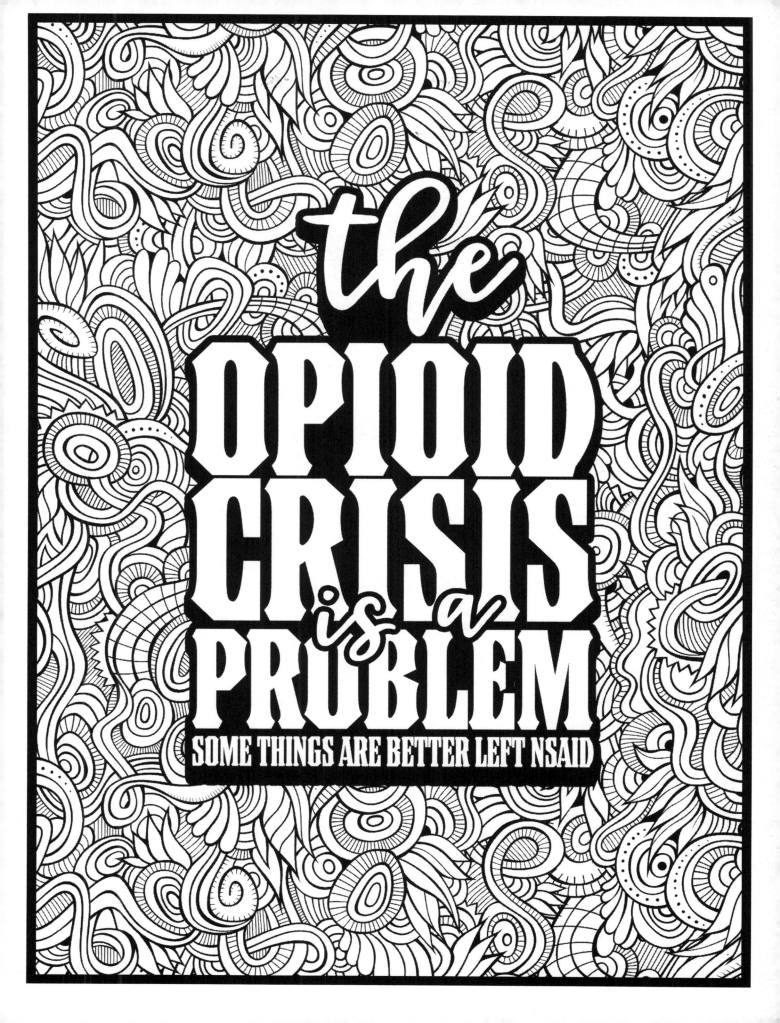

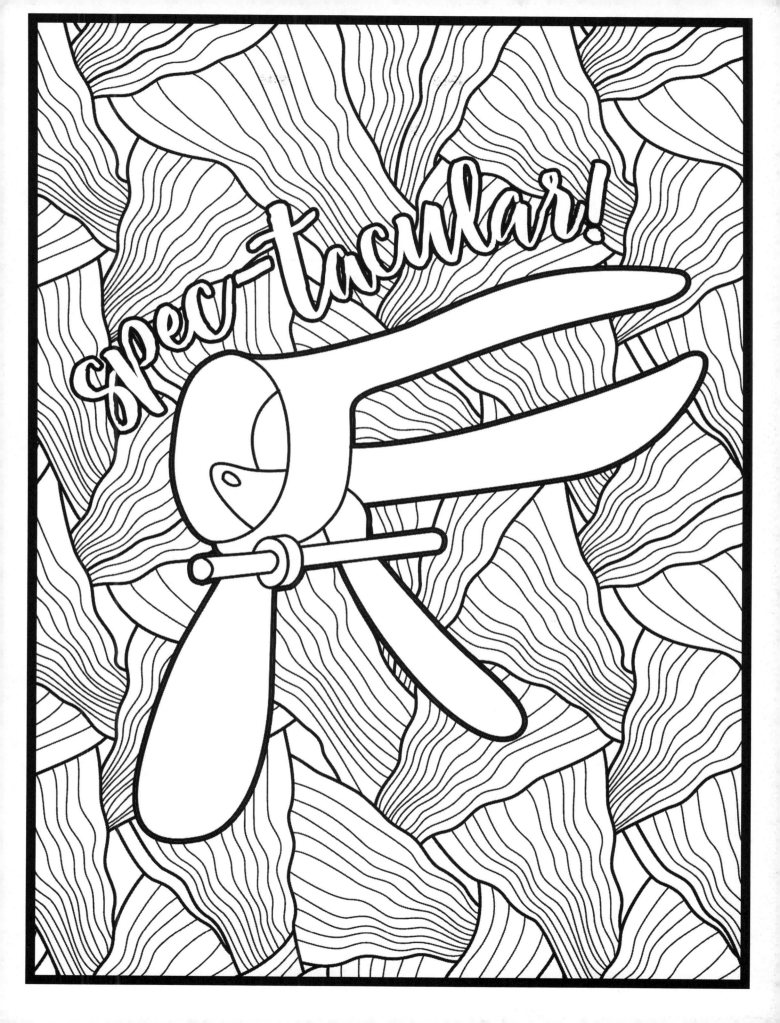

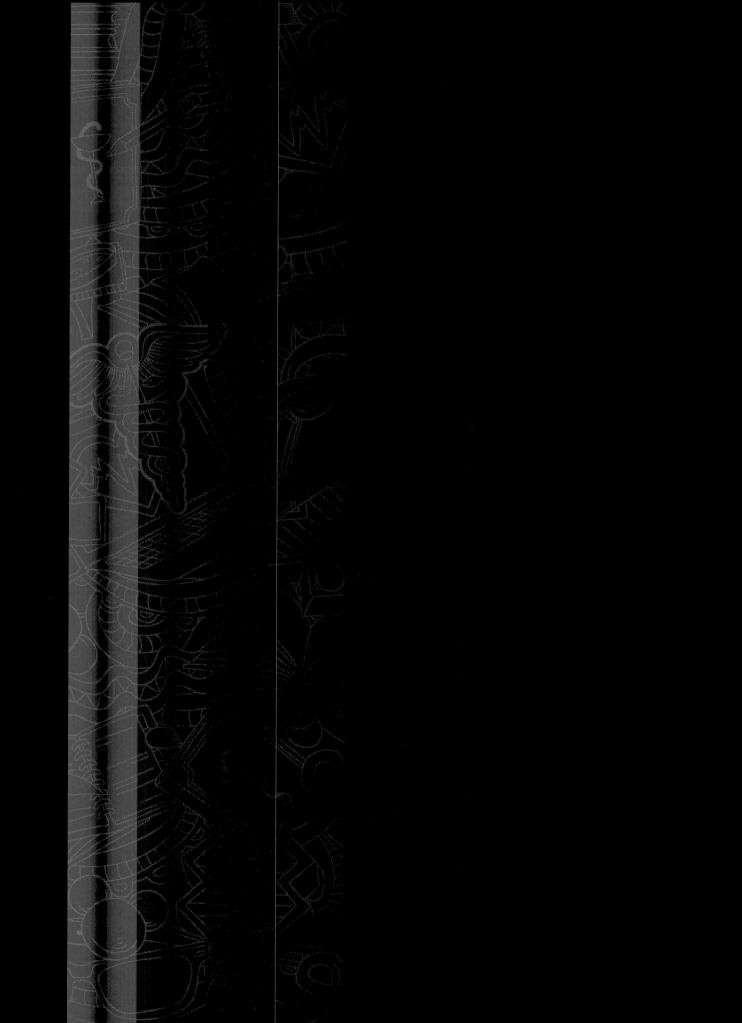

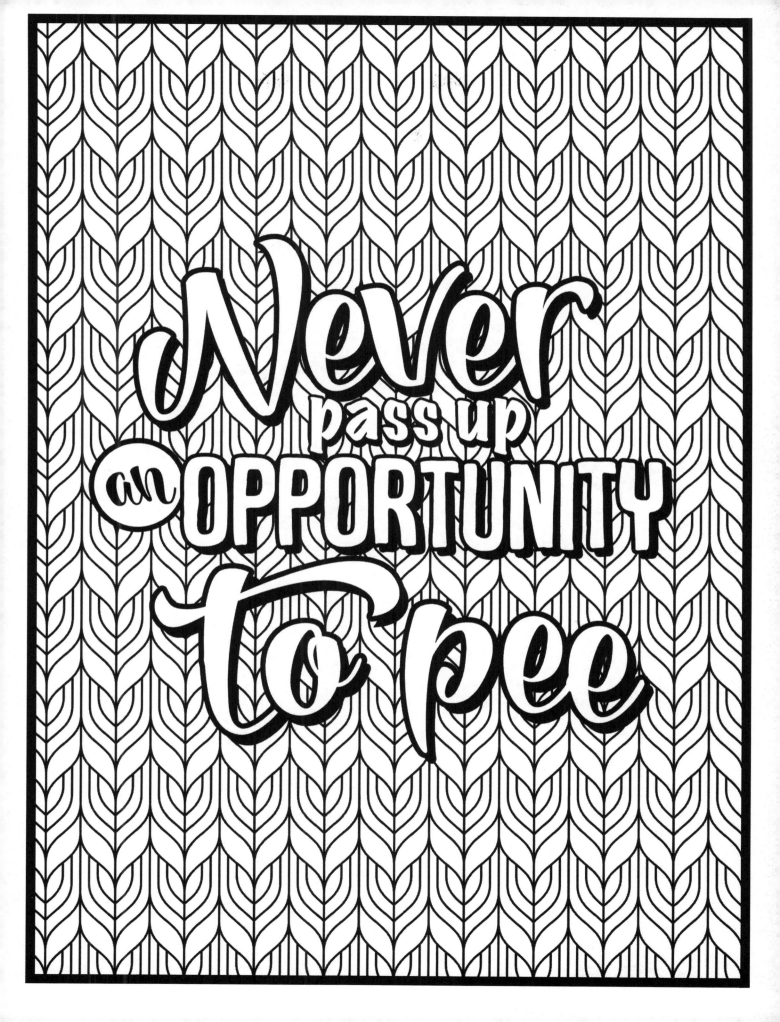

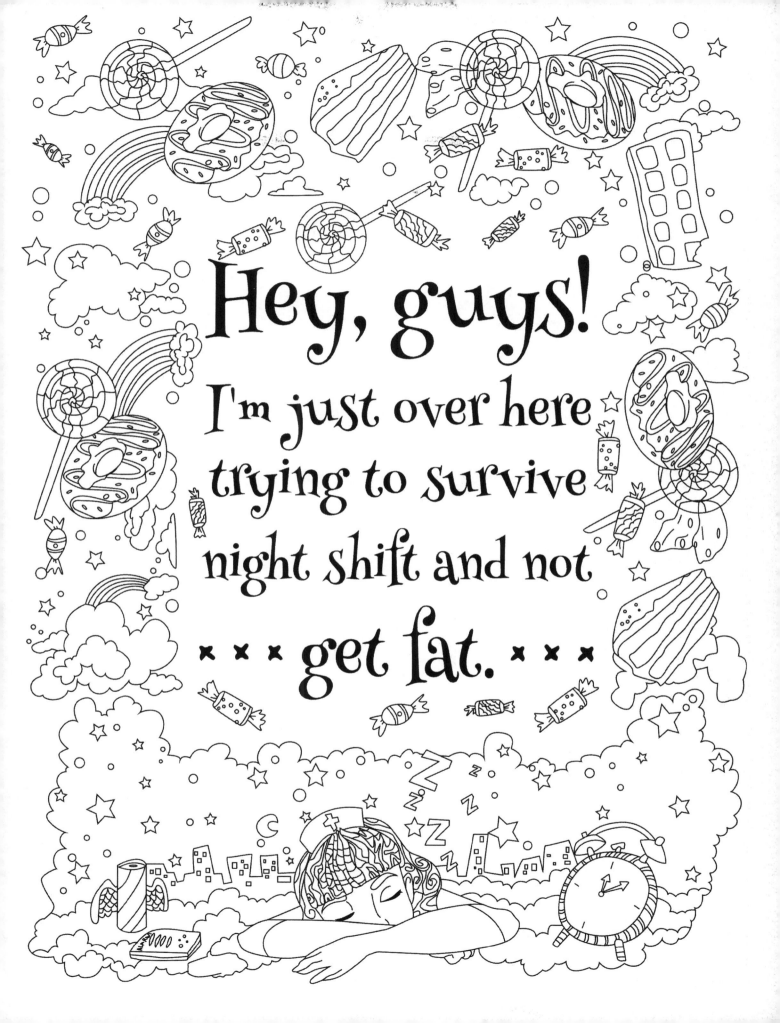

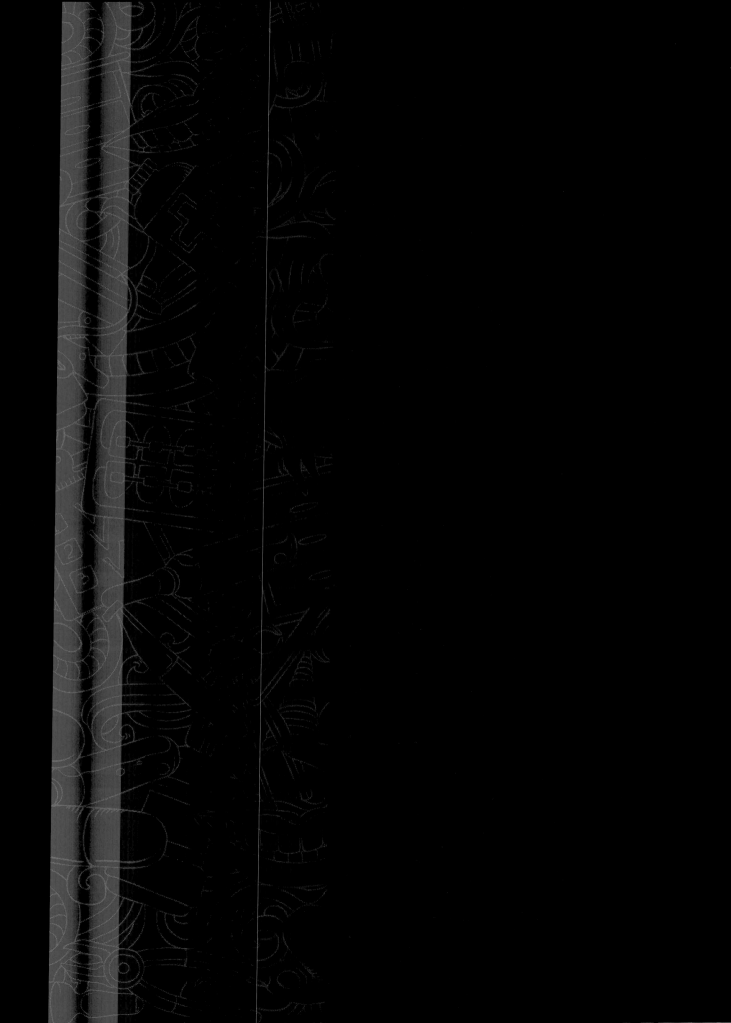

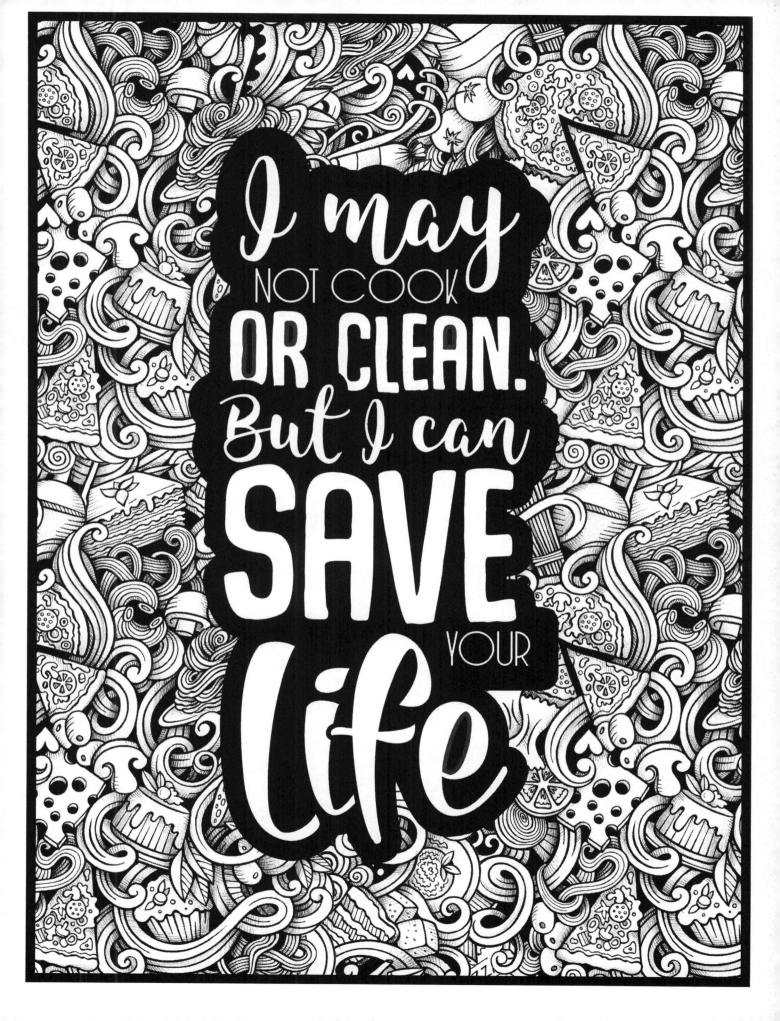

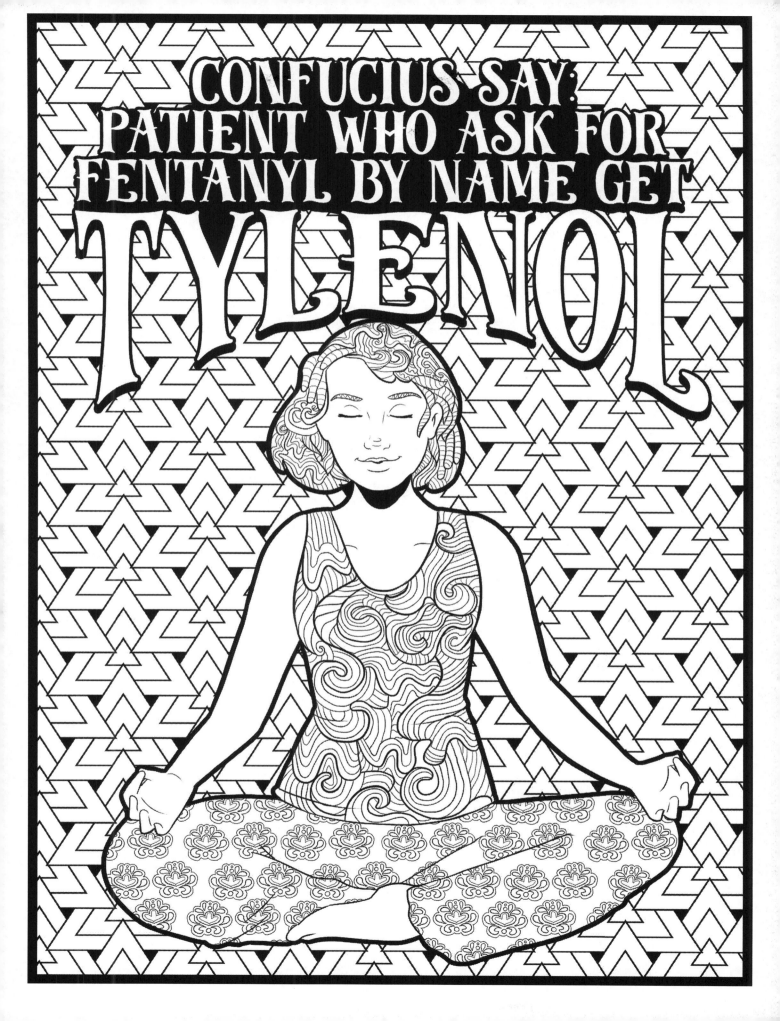

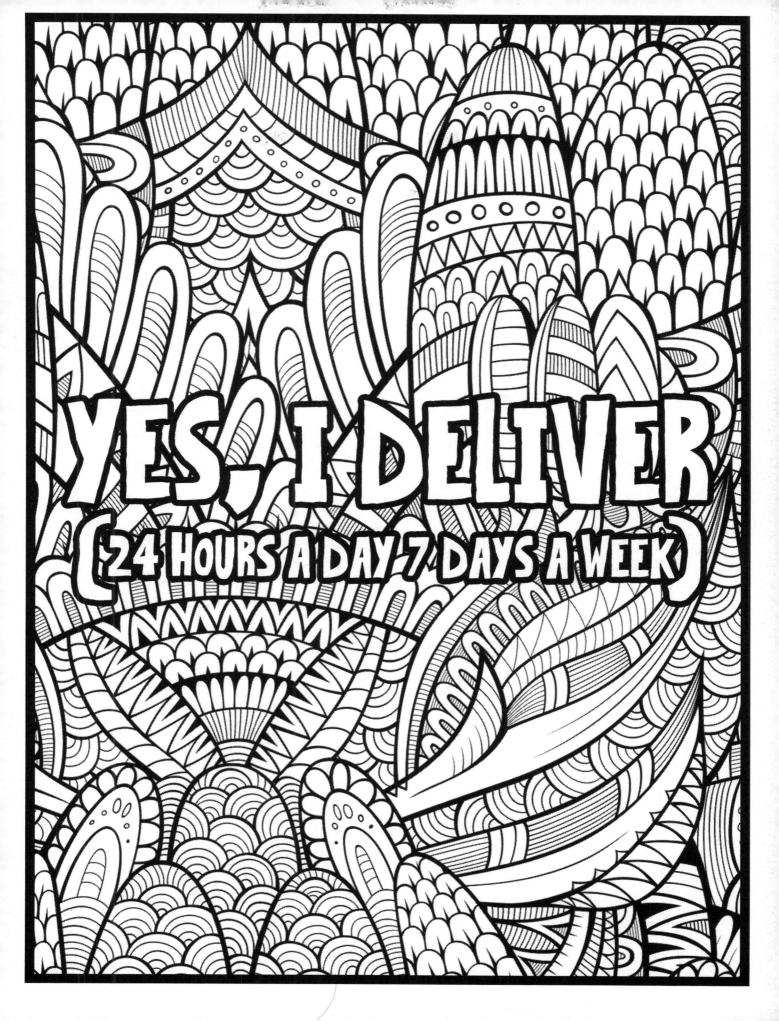

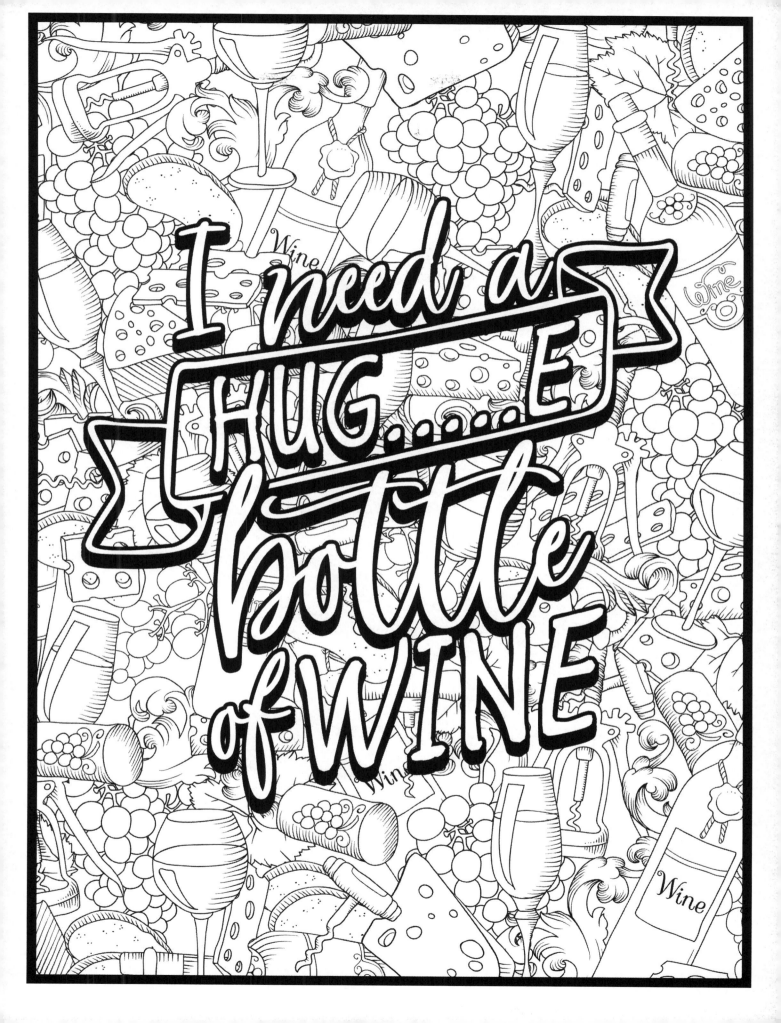

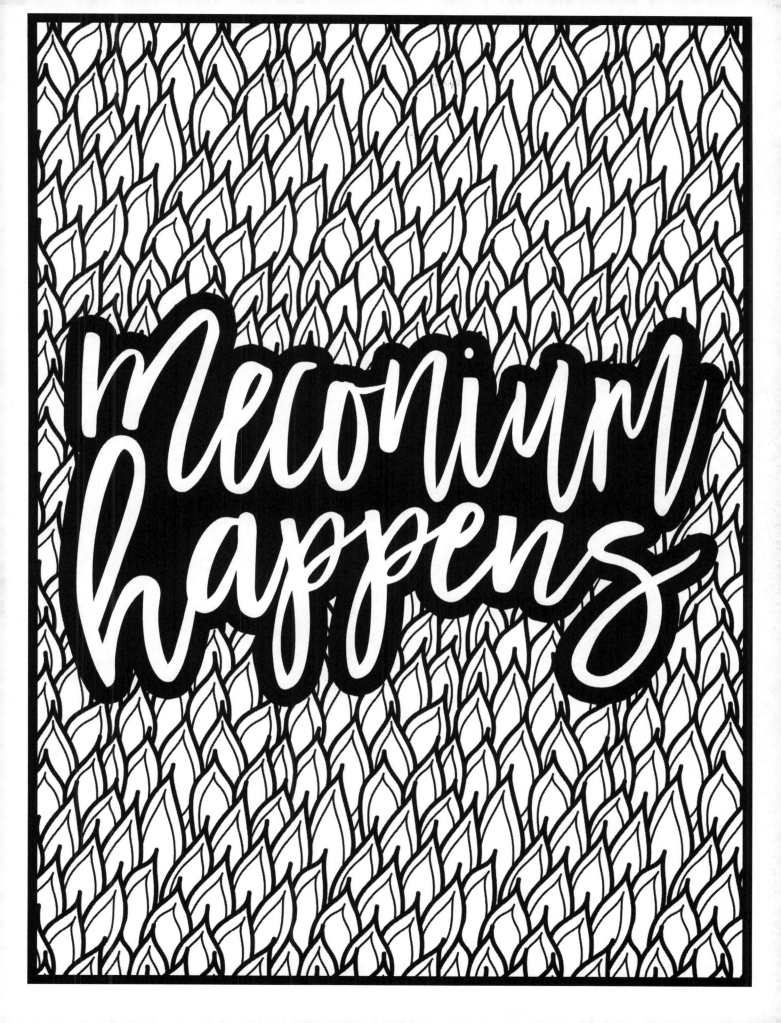

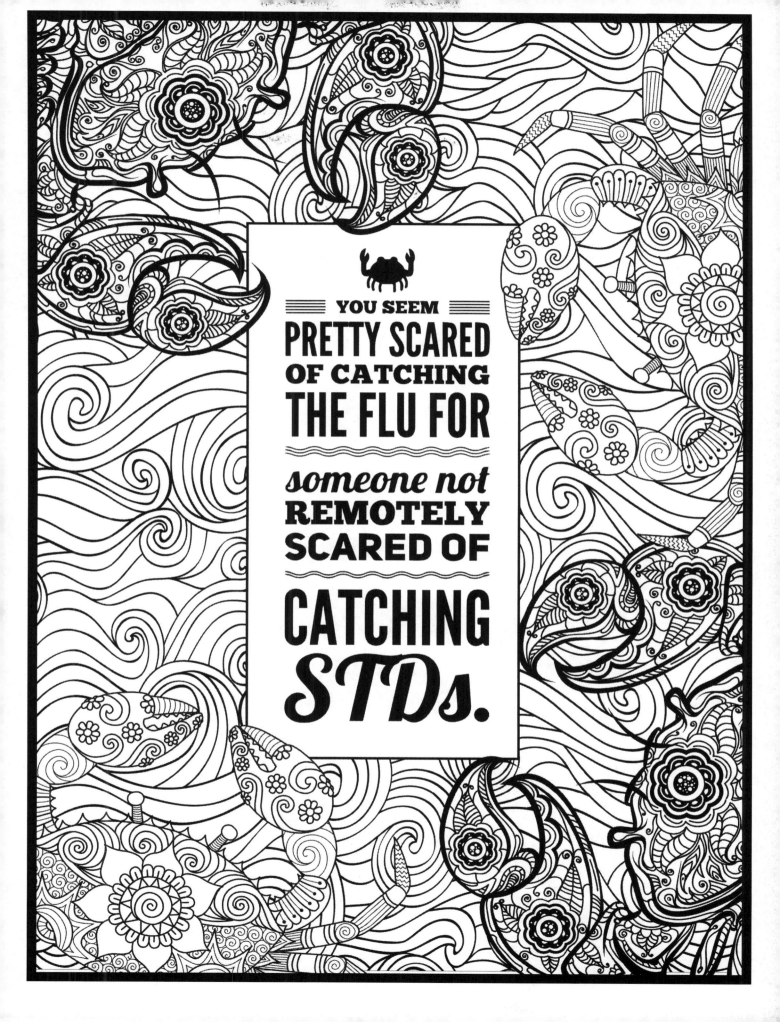

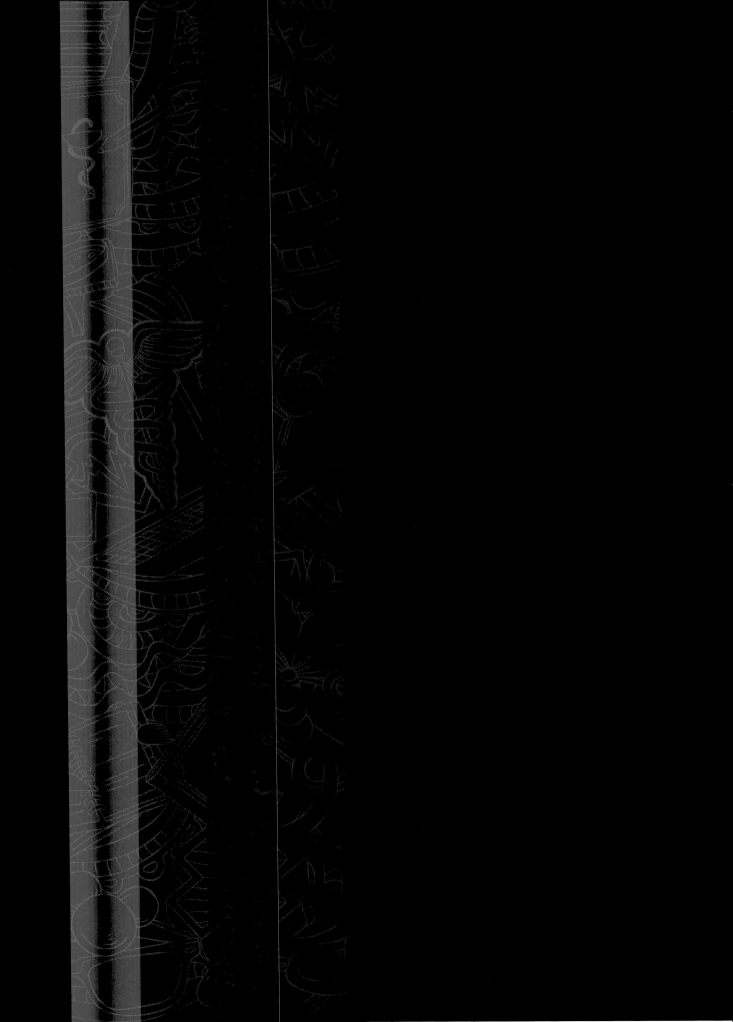

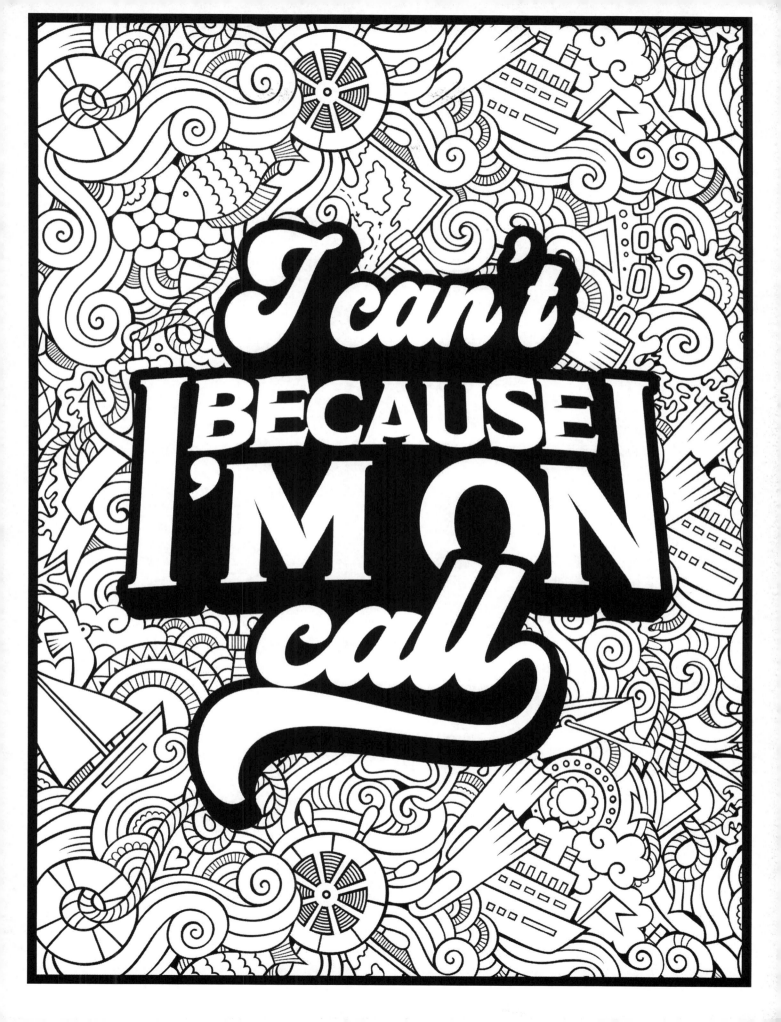

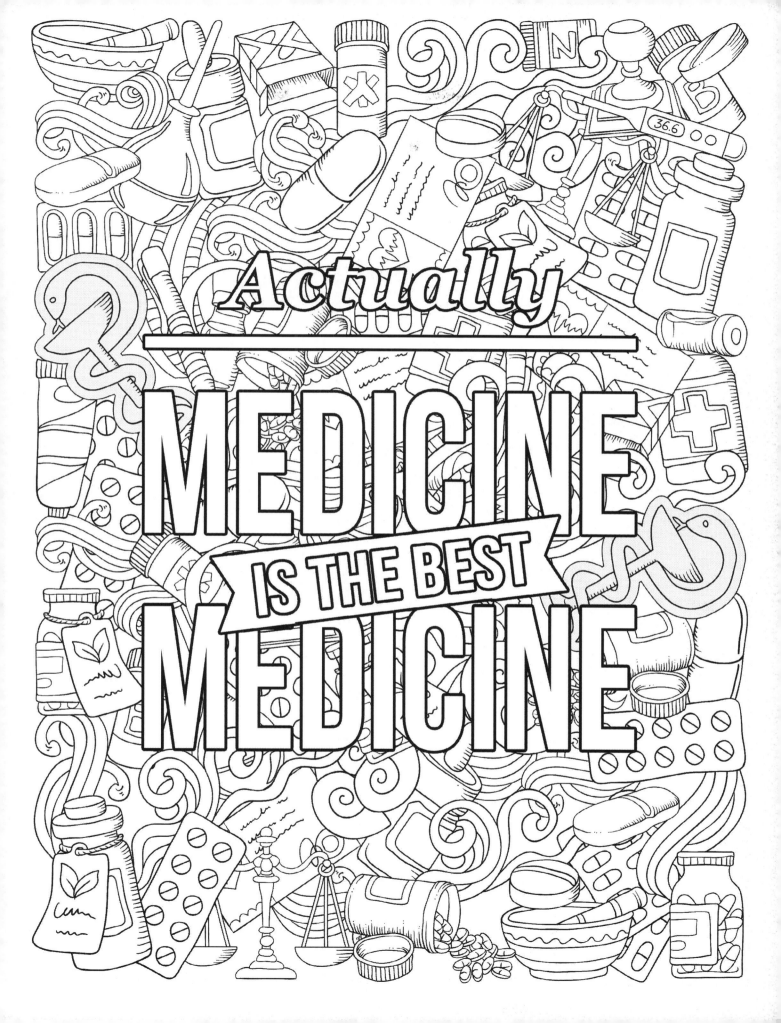

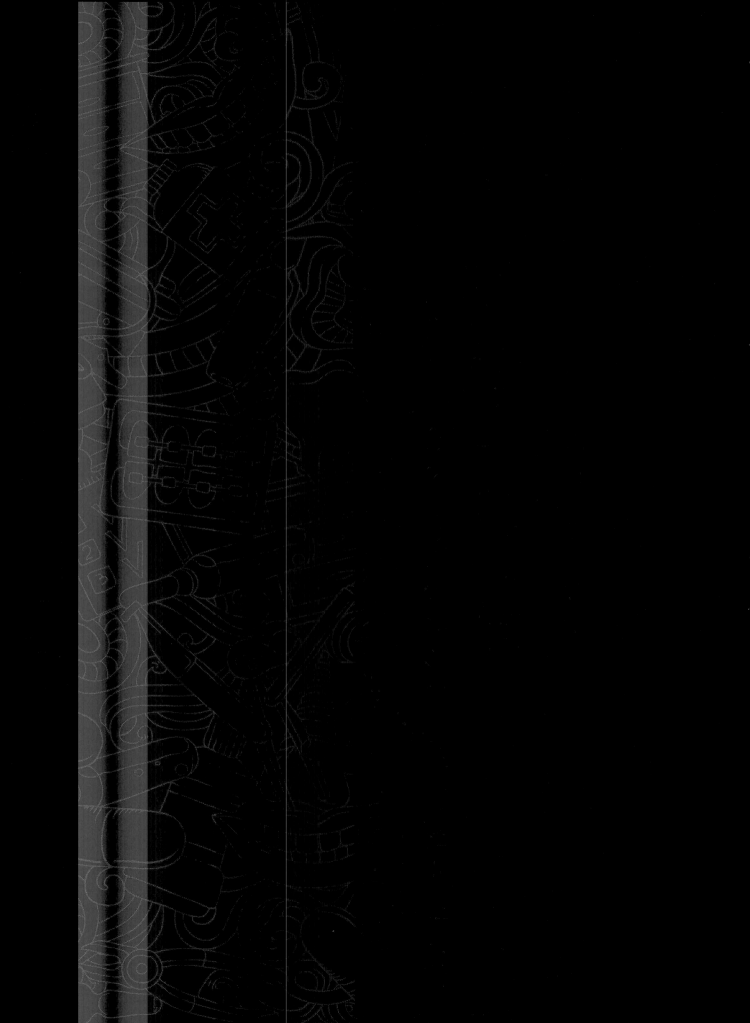

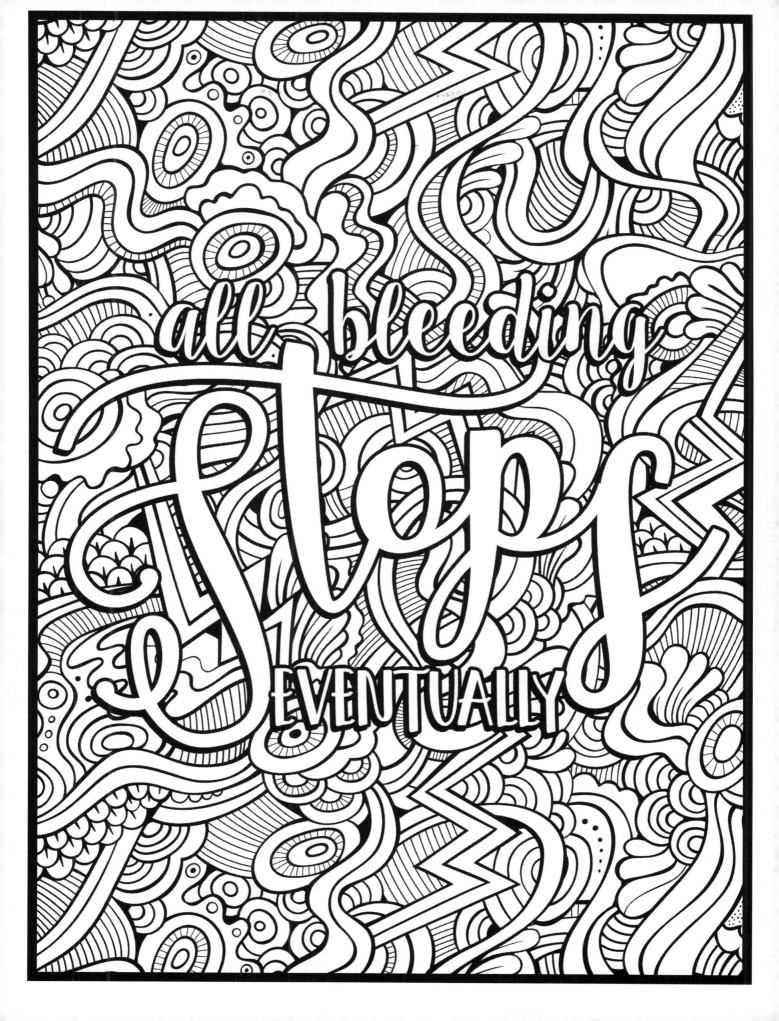

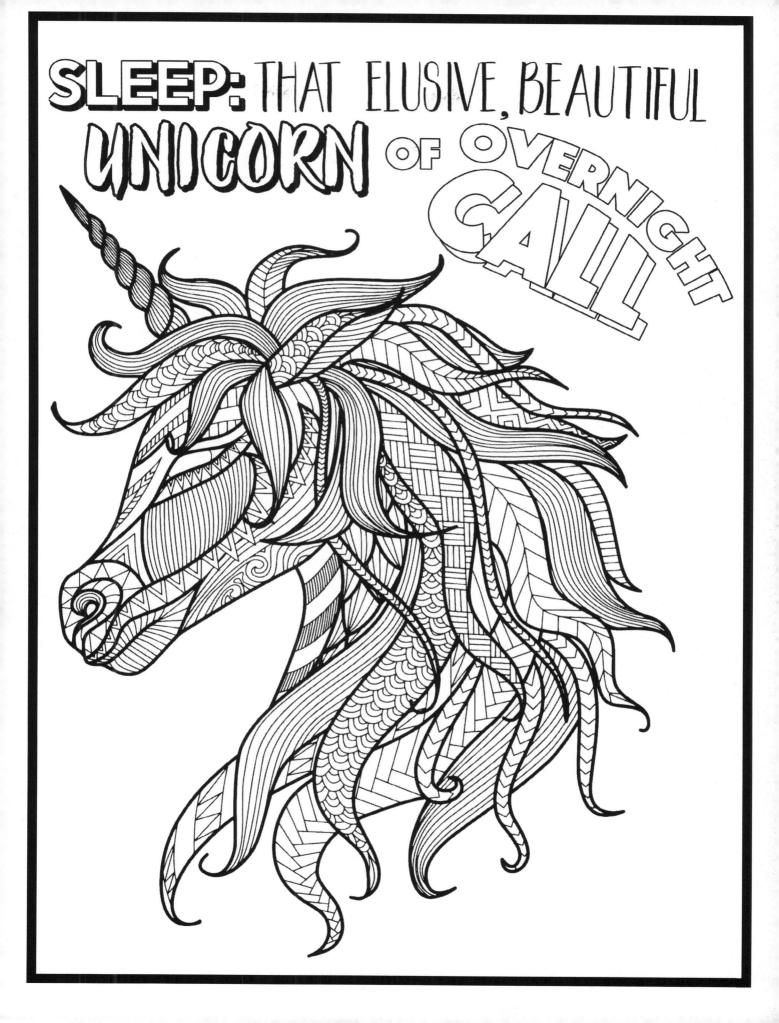

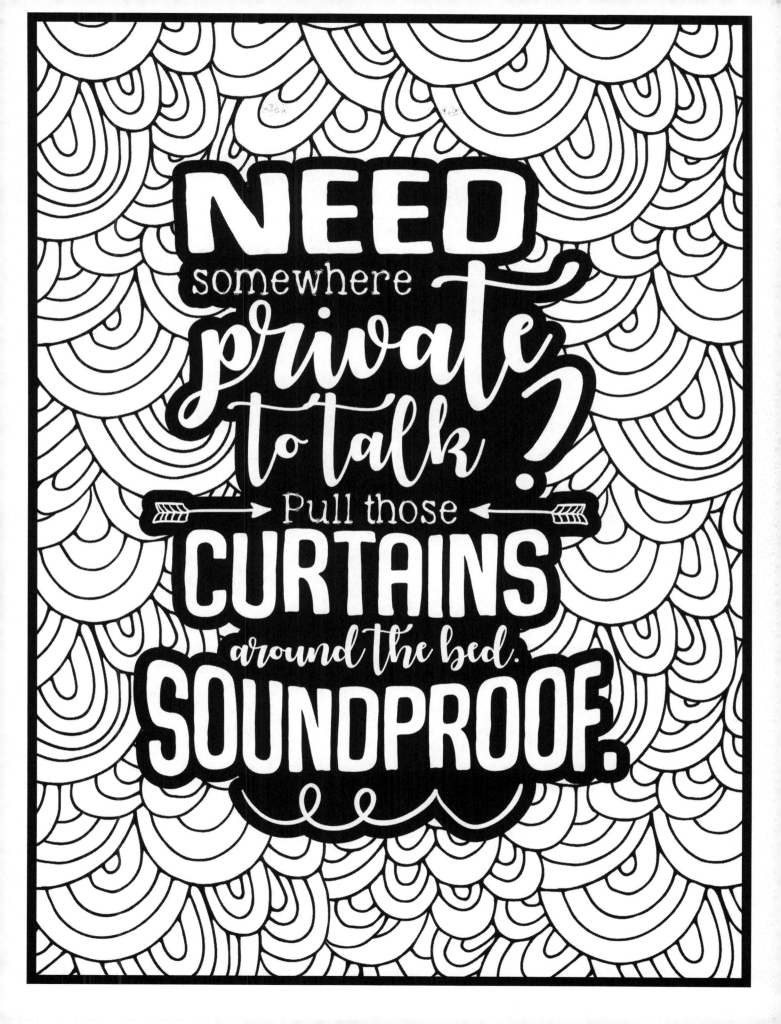

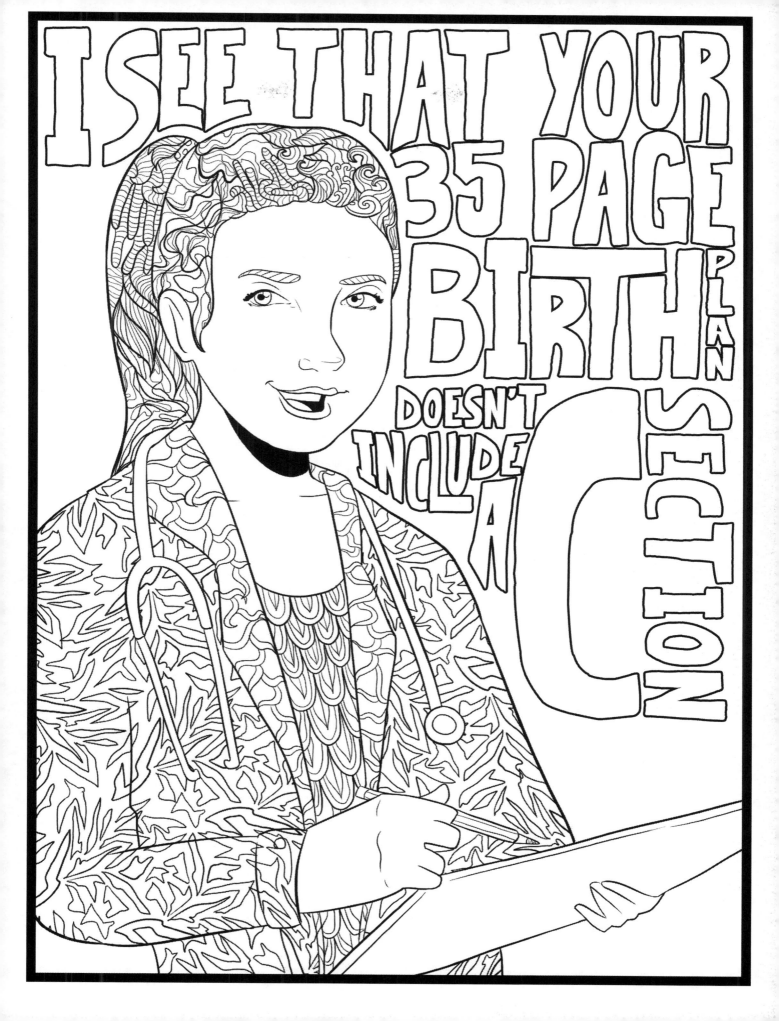

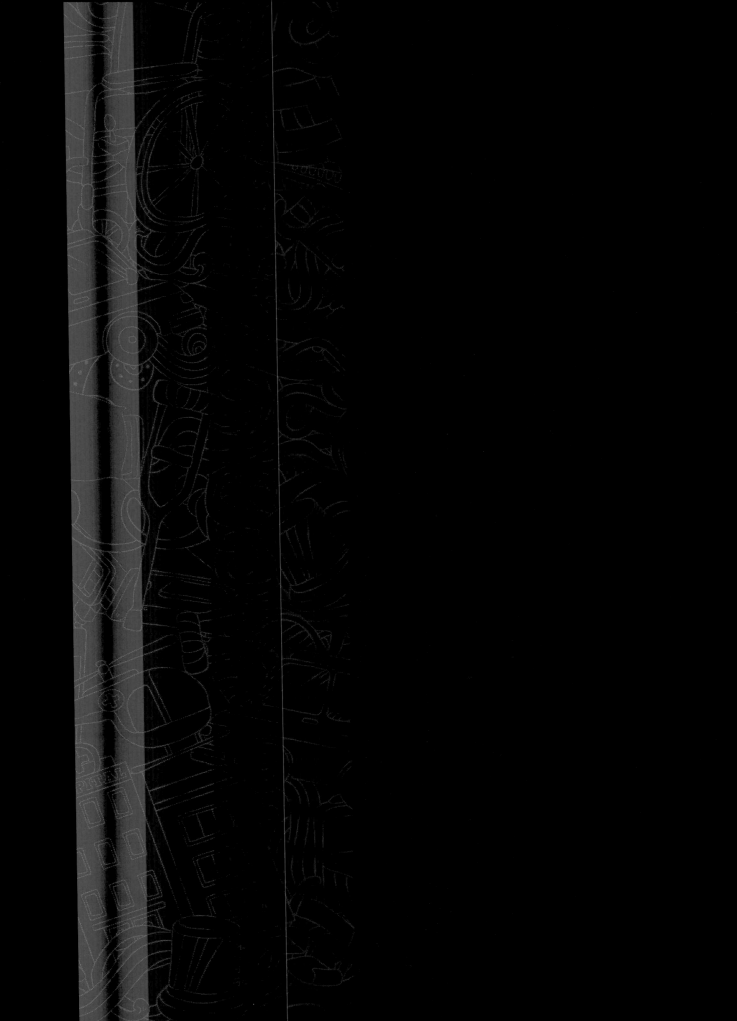

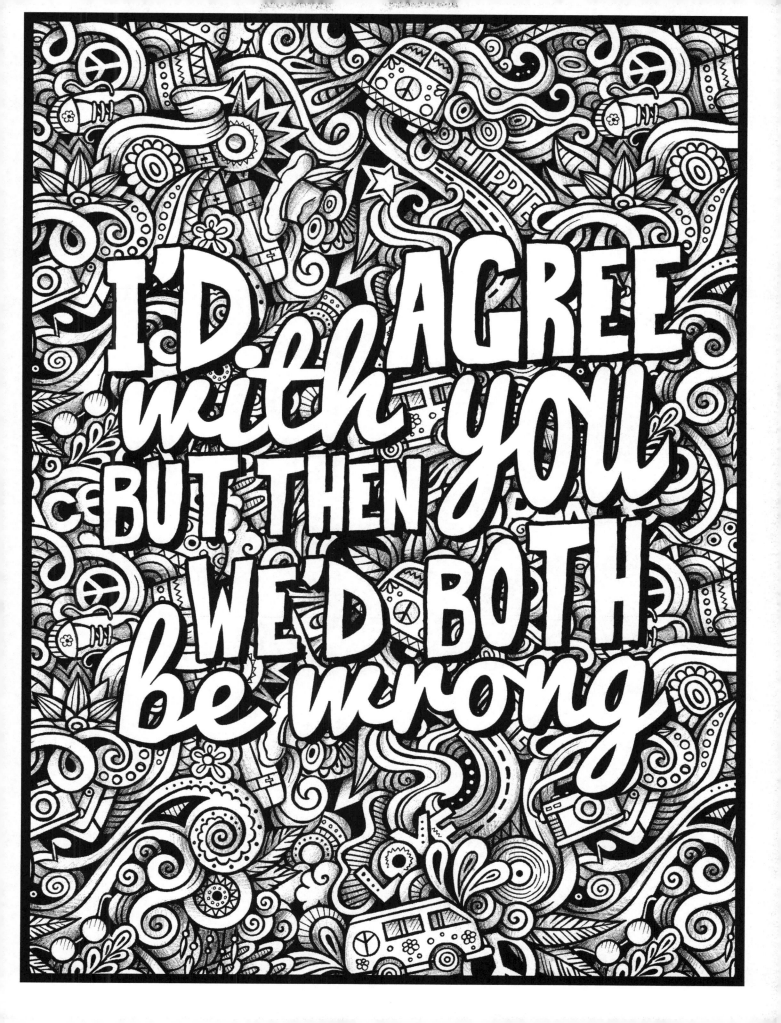

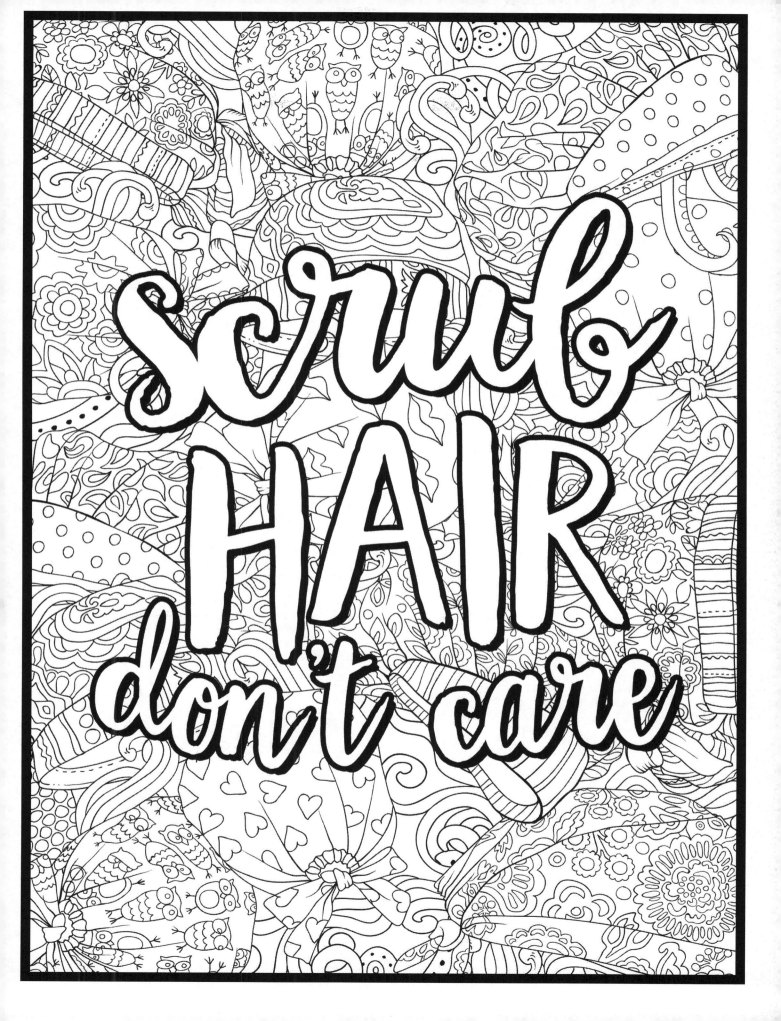

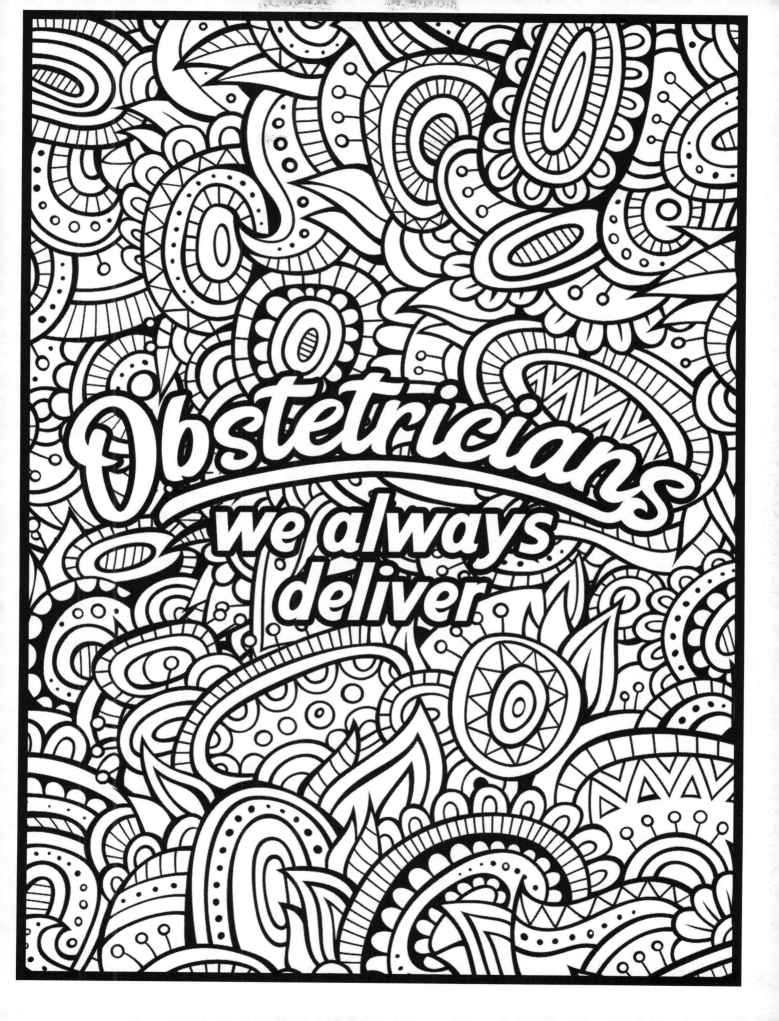

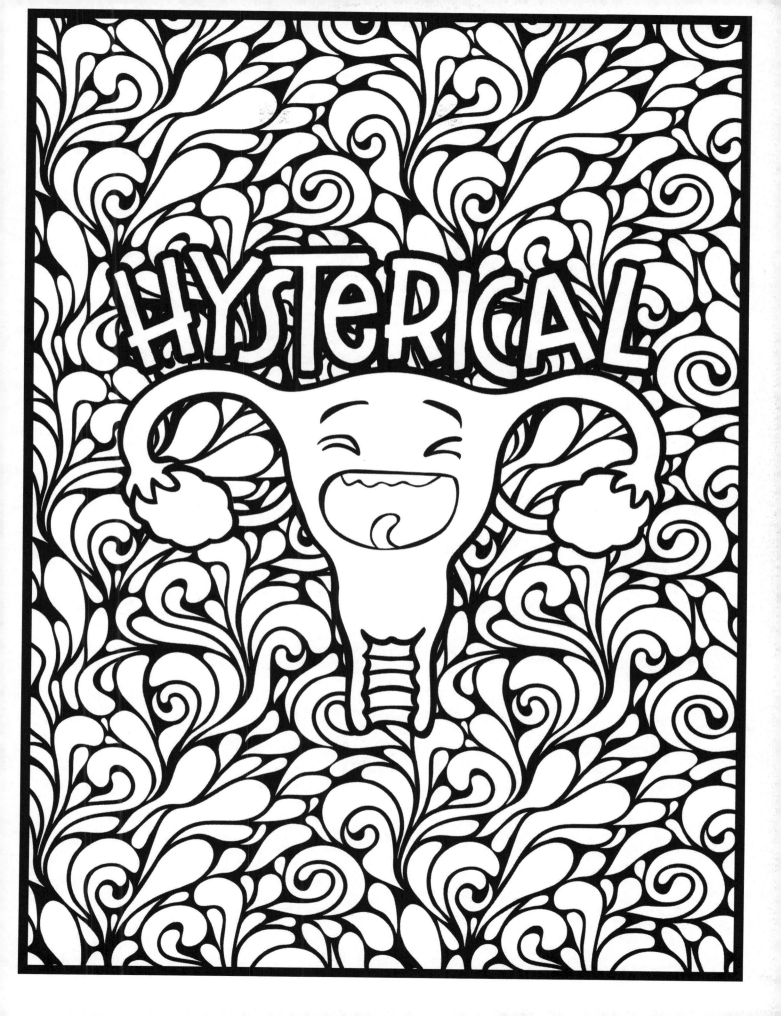

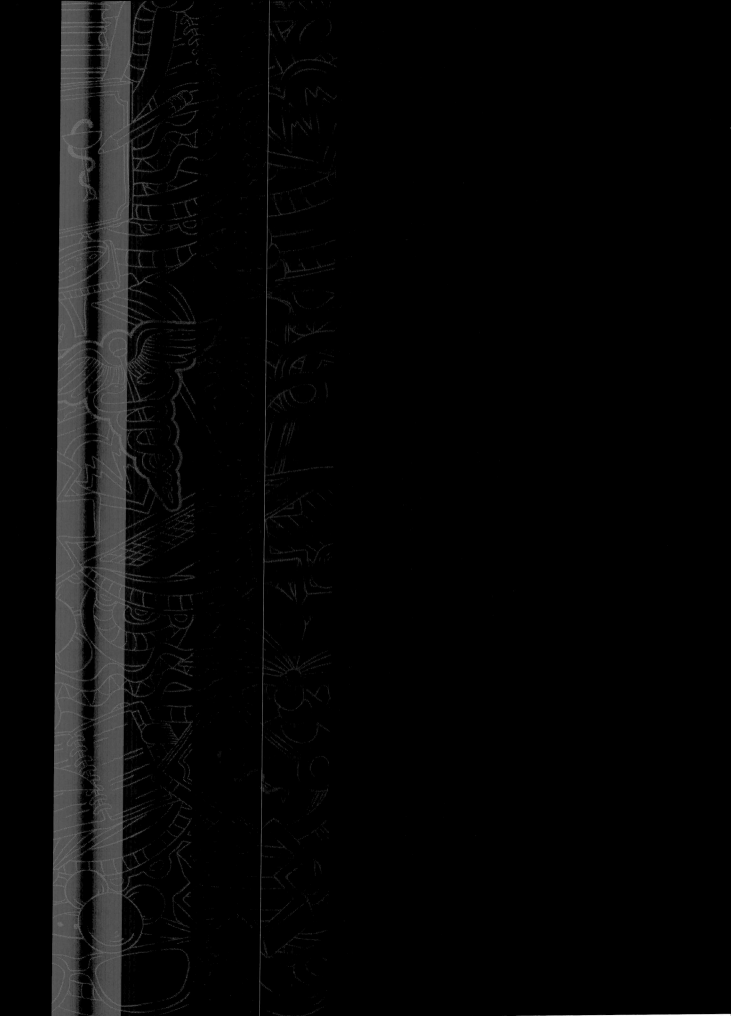

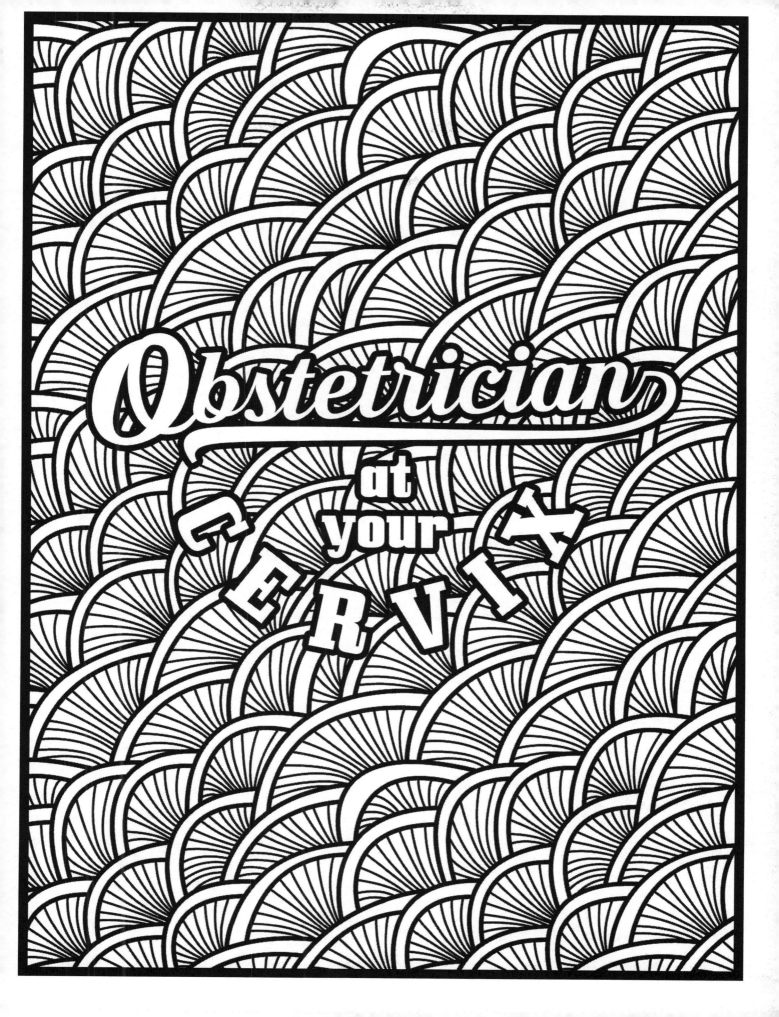

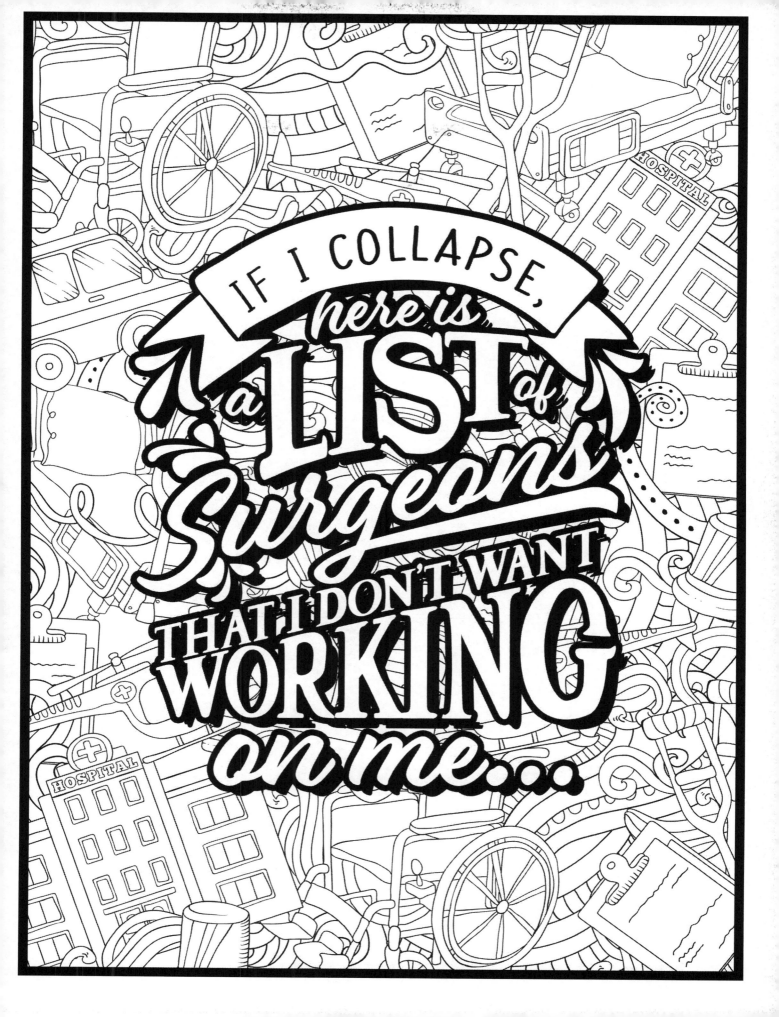

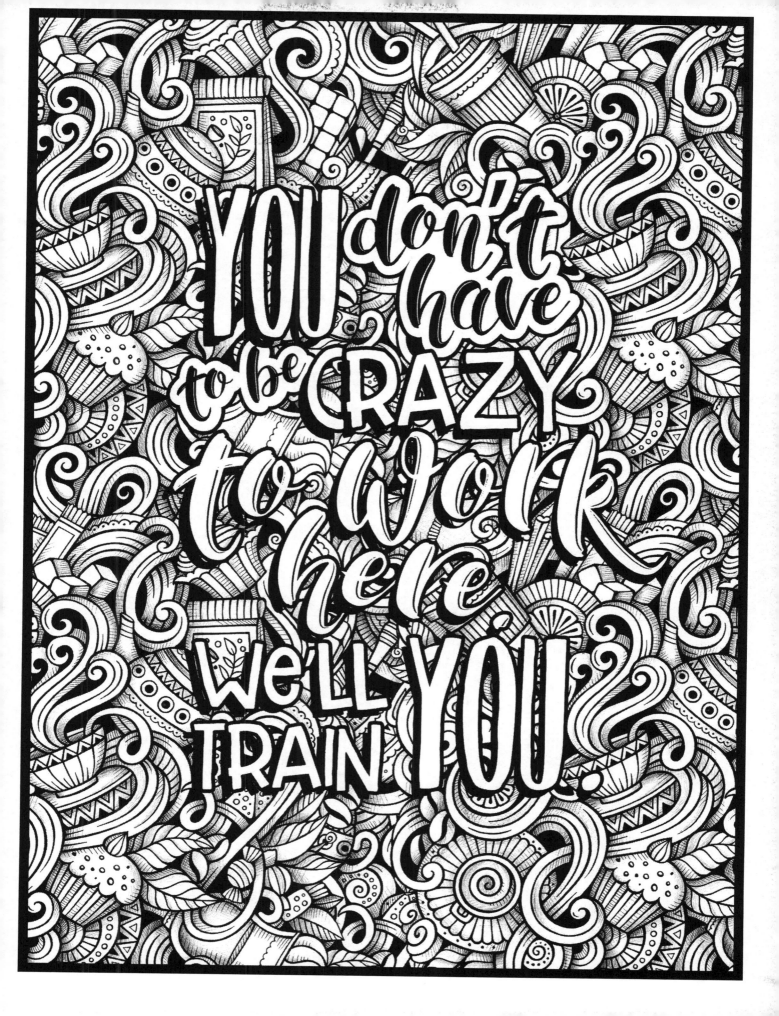

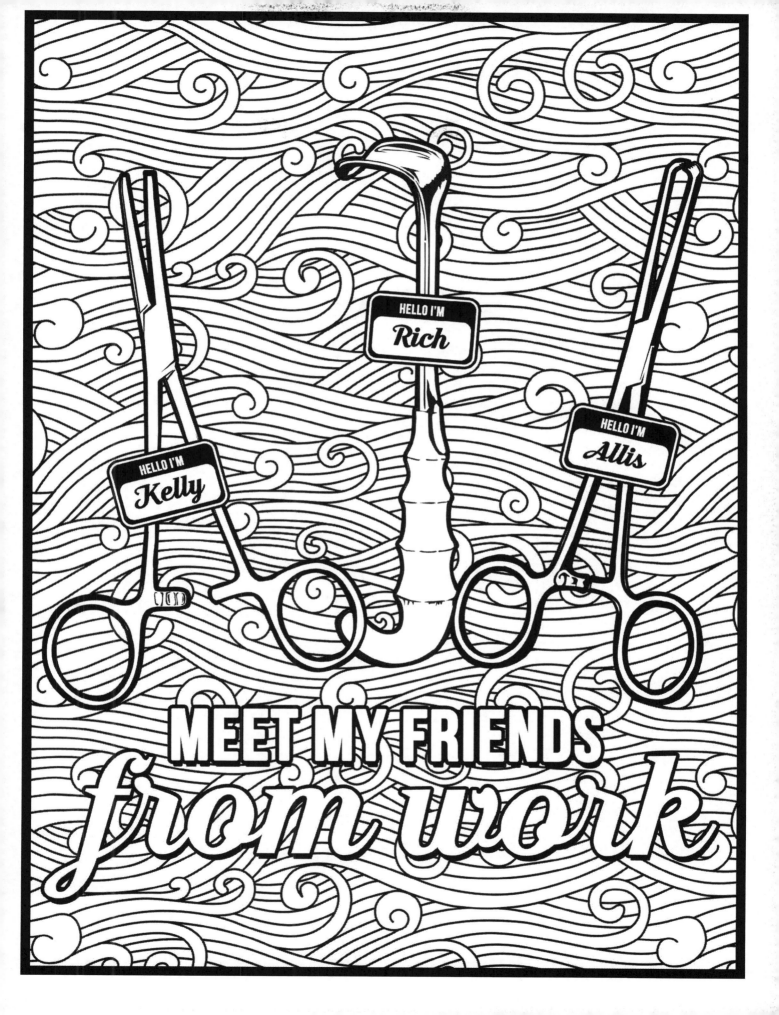

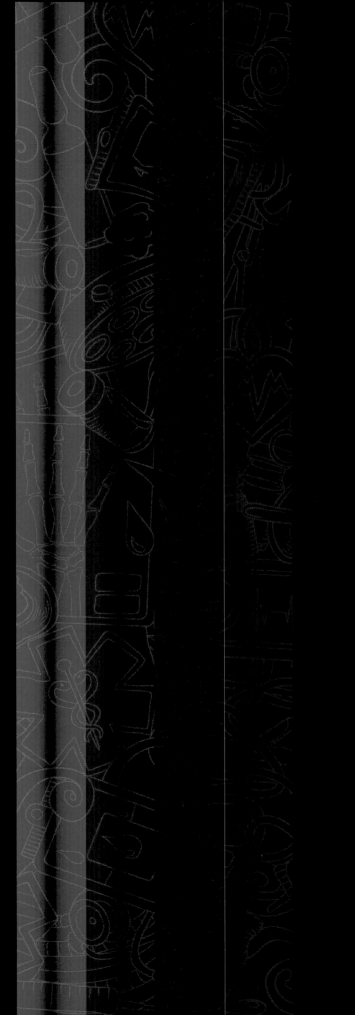

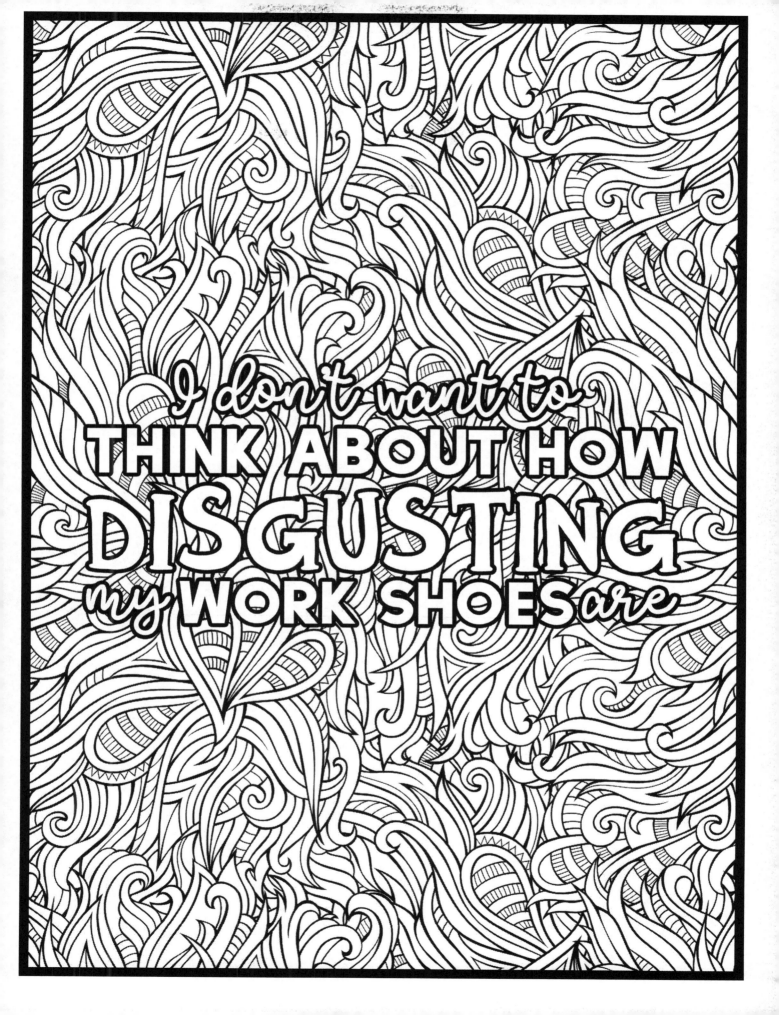

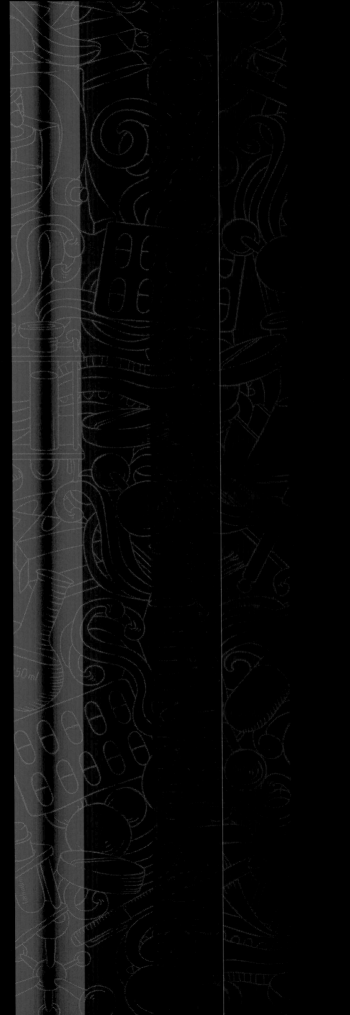

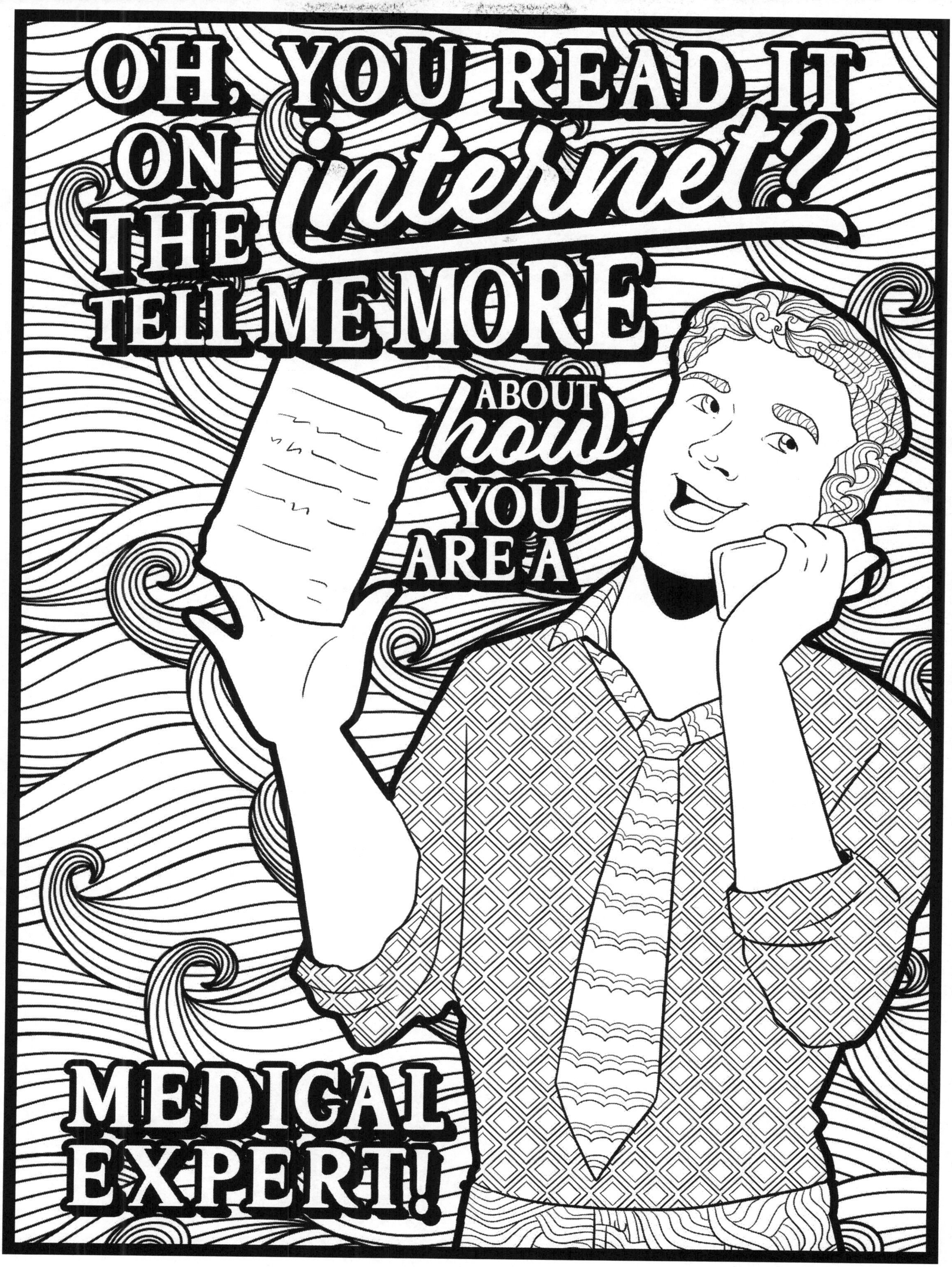
OH, YOU READ IT
ON
THE internet?
TELL ME MORE
ABOUT
how
YOU
ARE A
MEDICAL
EXPERT!

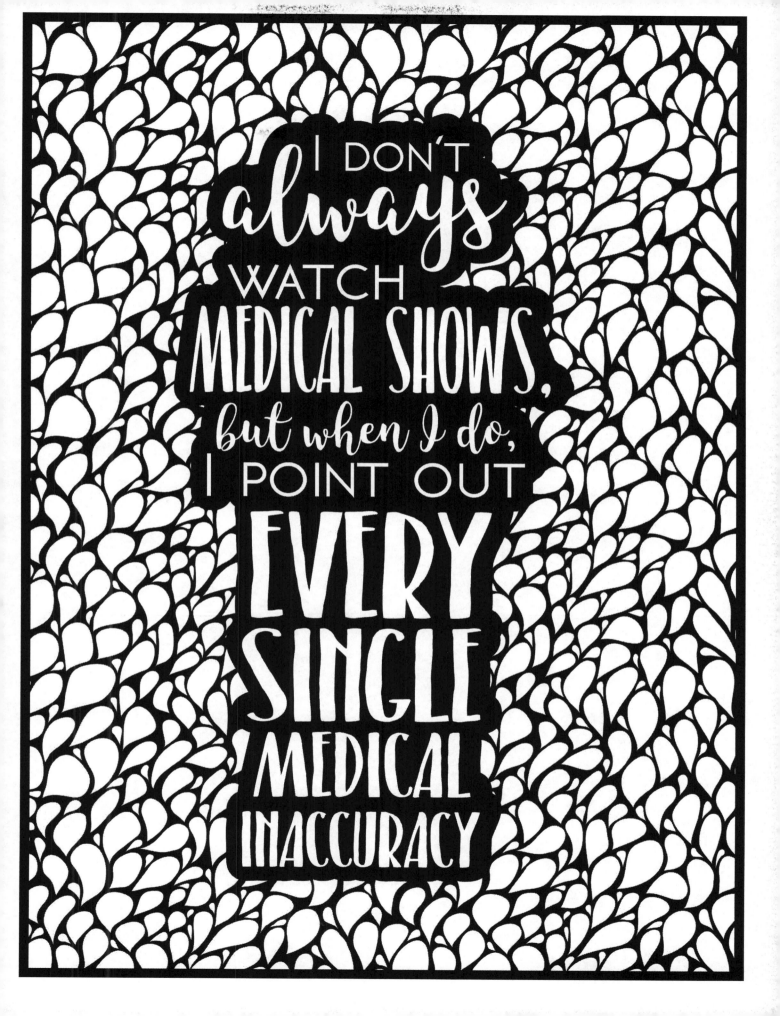

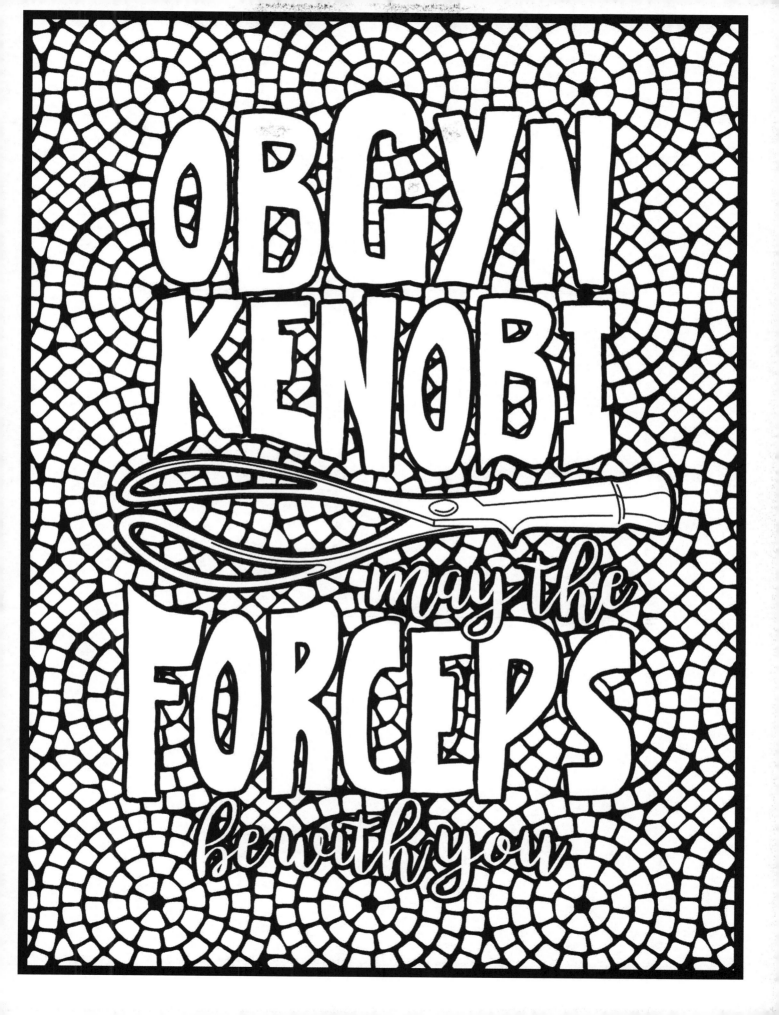

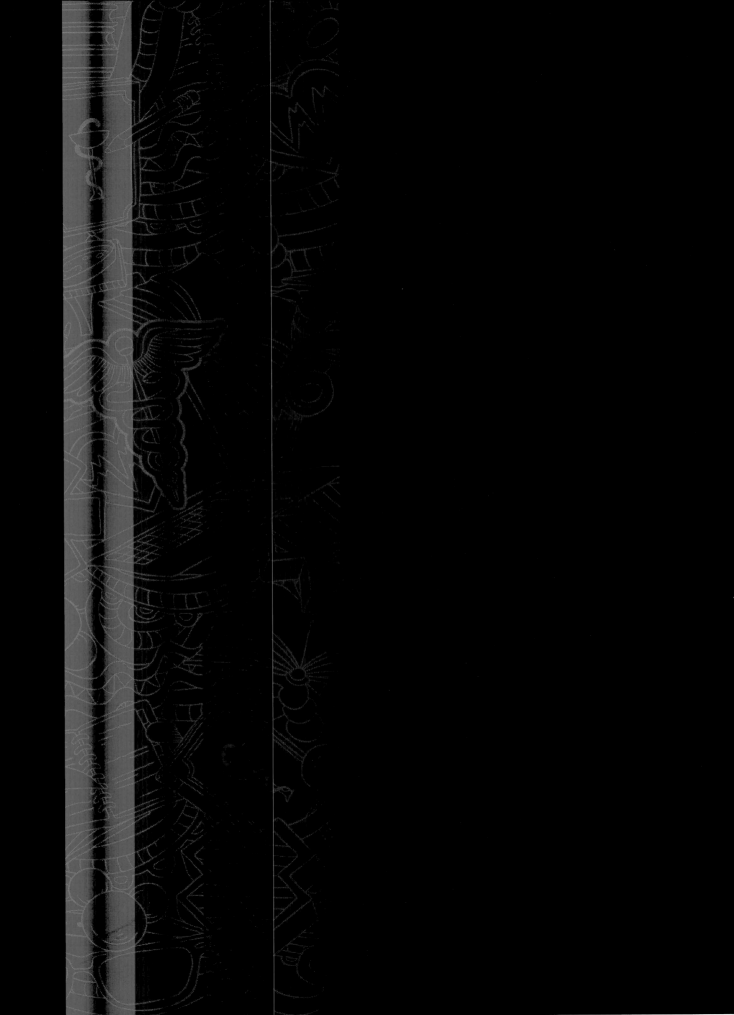

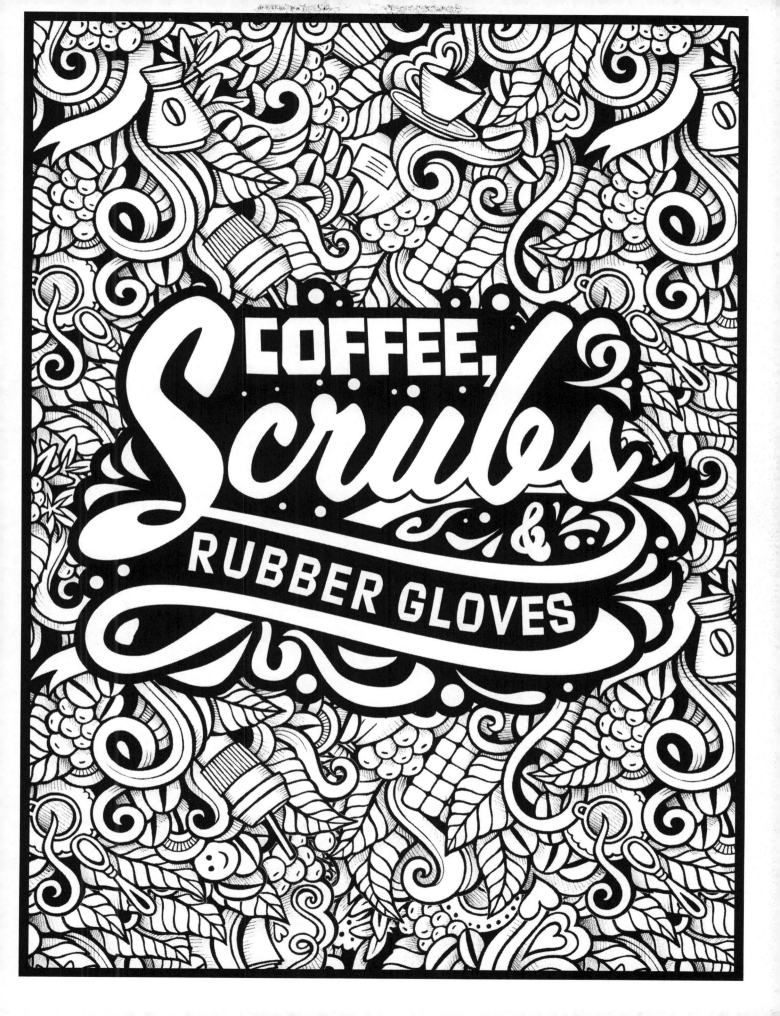

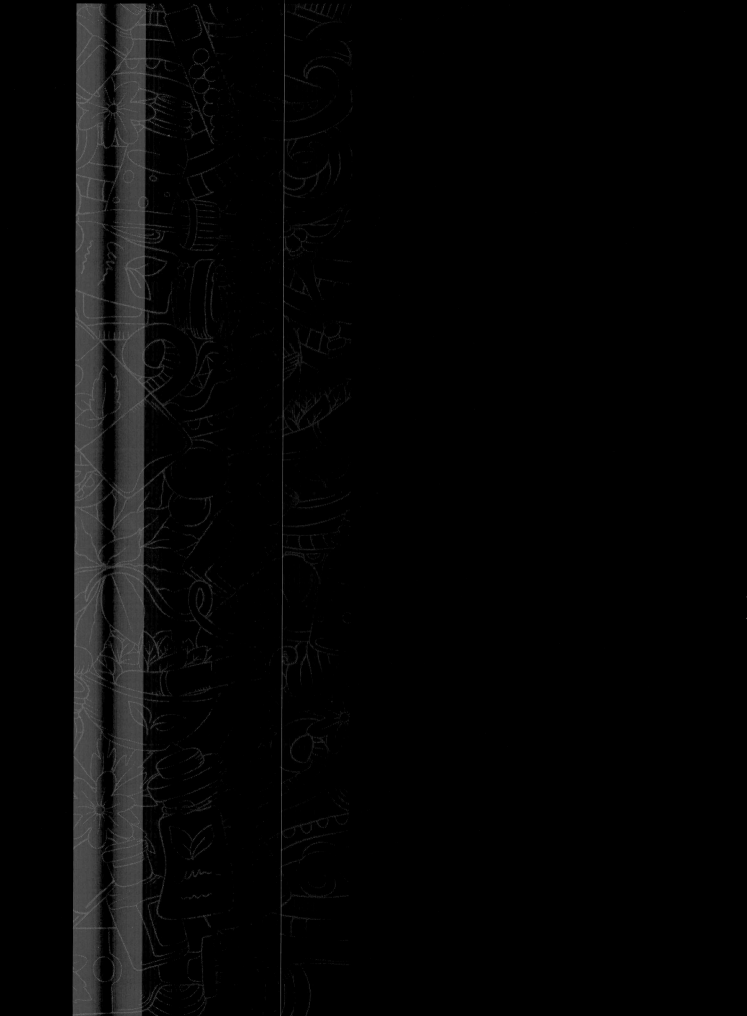

SORRY, BUT YOUR PASSWORD MUST CONTAIN A SYMBOL. A NUMBER. AN UPPERCASE LETTER. A HIEROGLYPH. A HAIKU. and THE BLOOD OF a VIRGIN

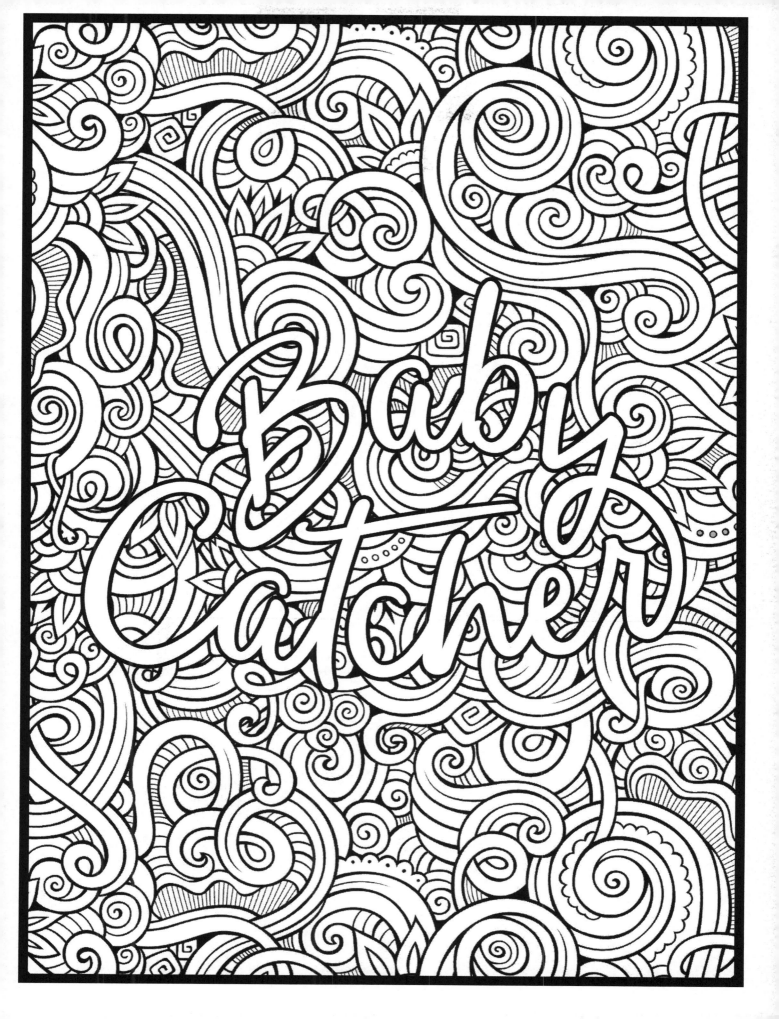

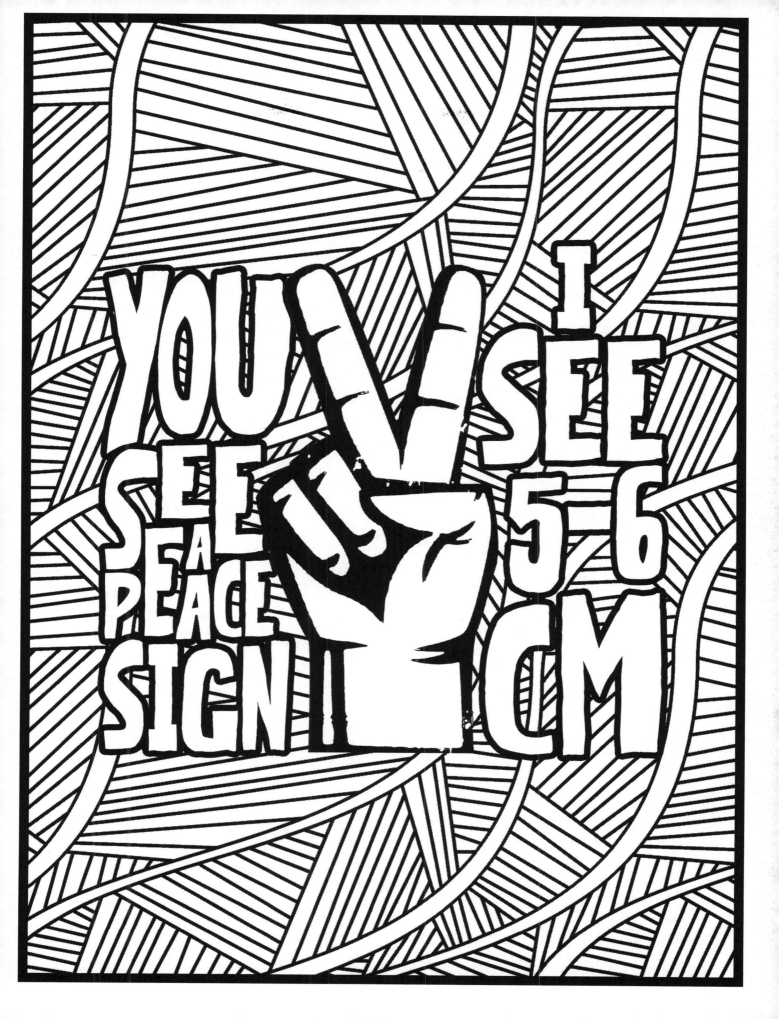

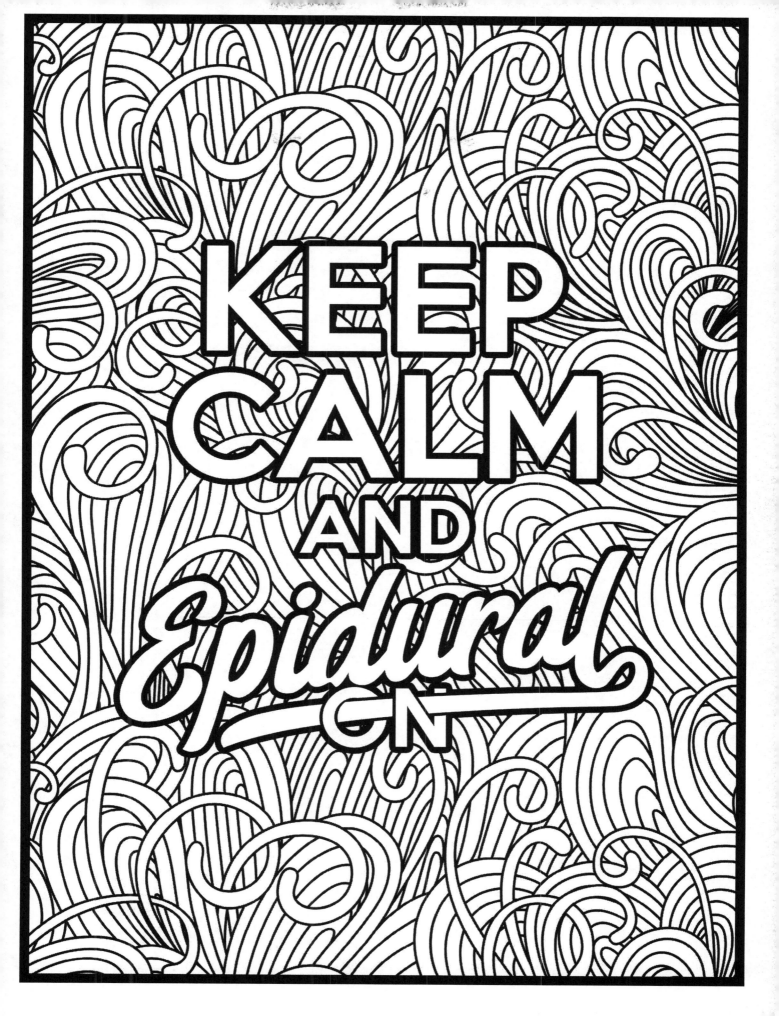

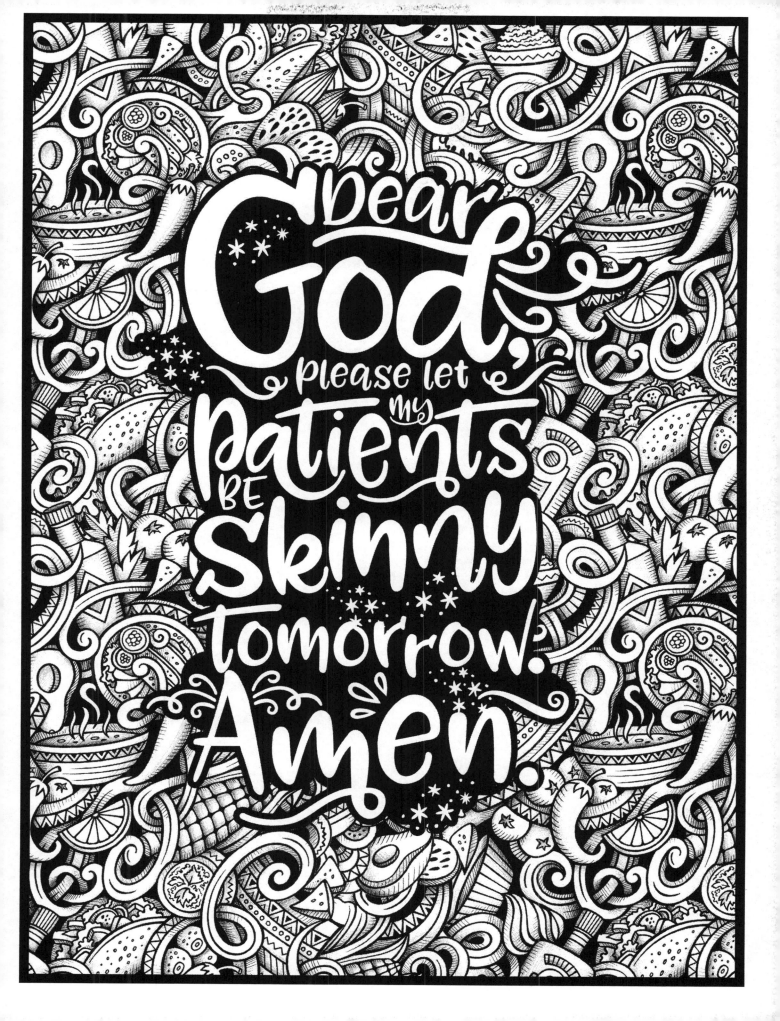

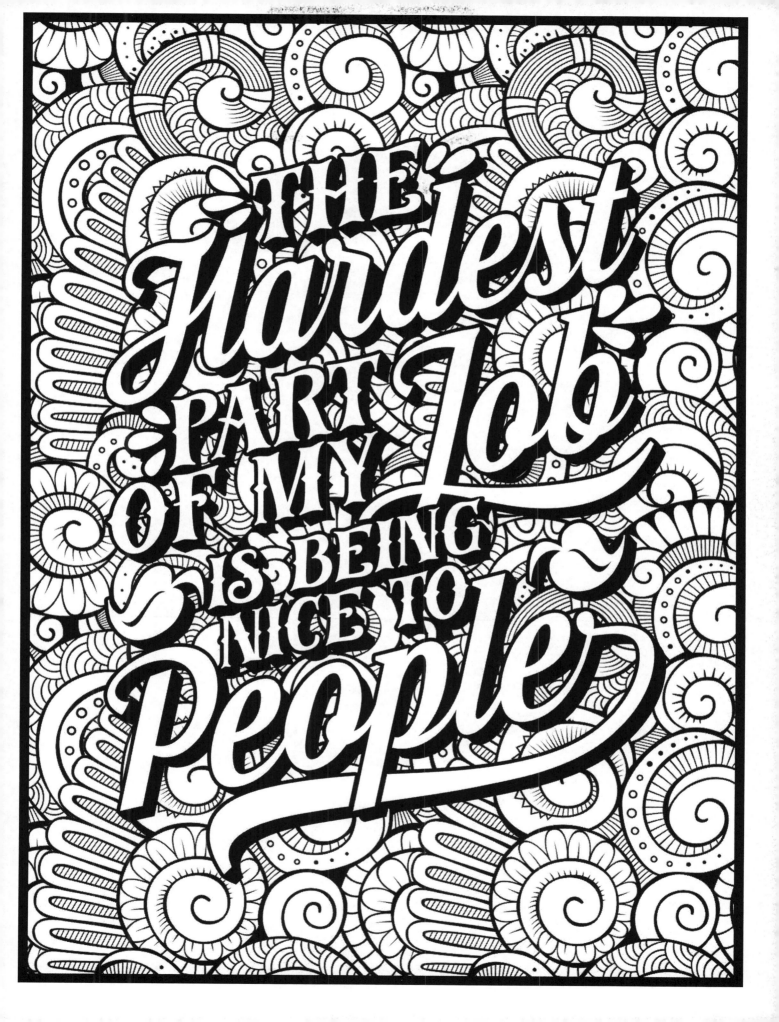

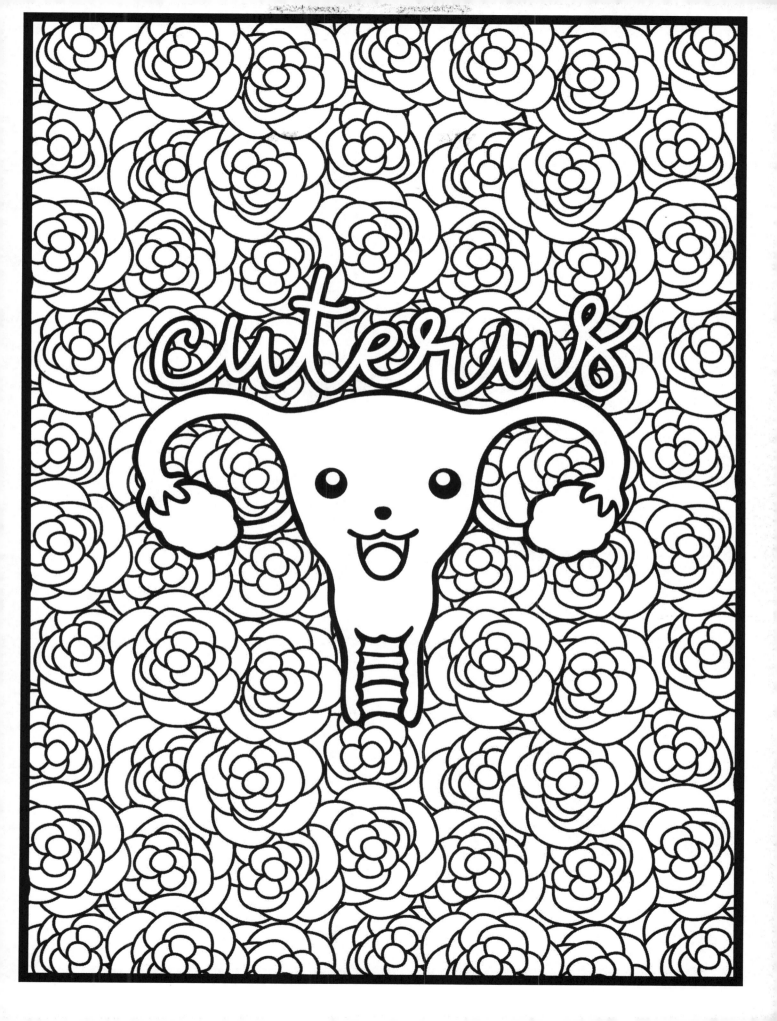

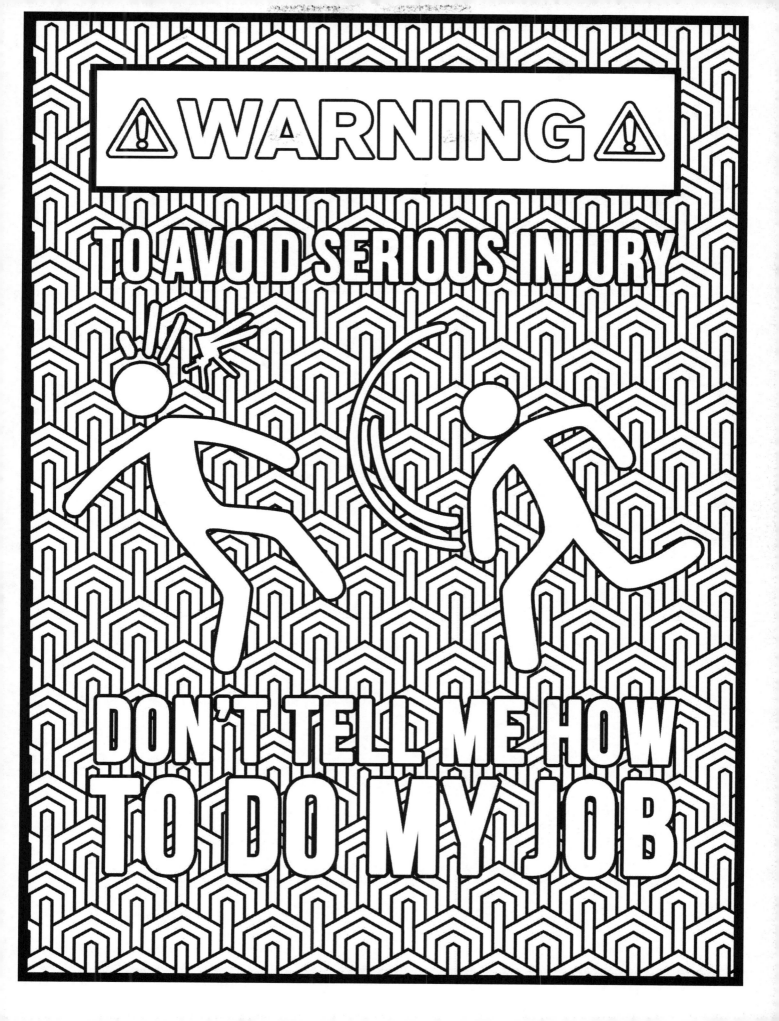

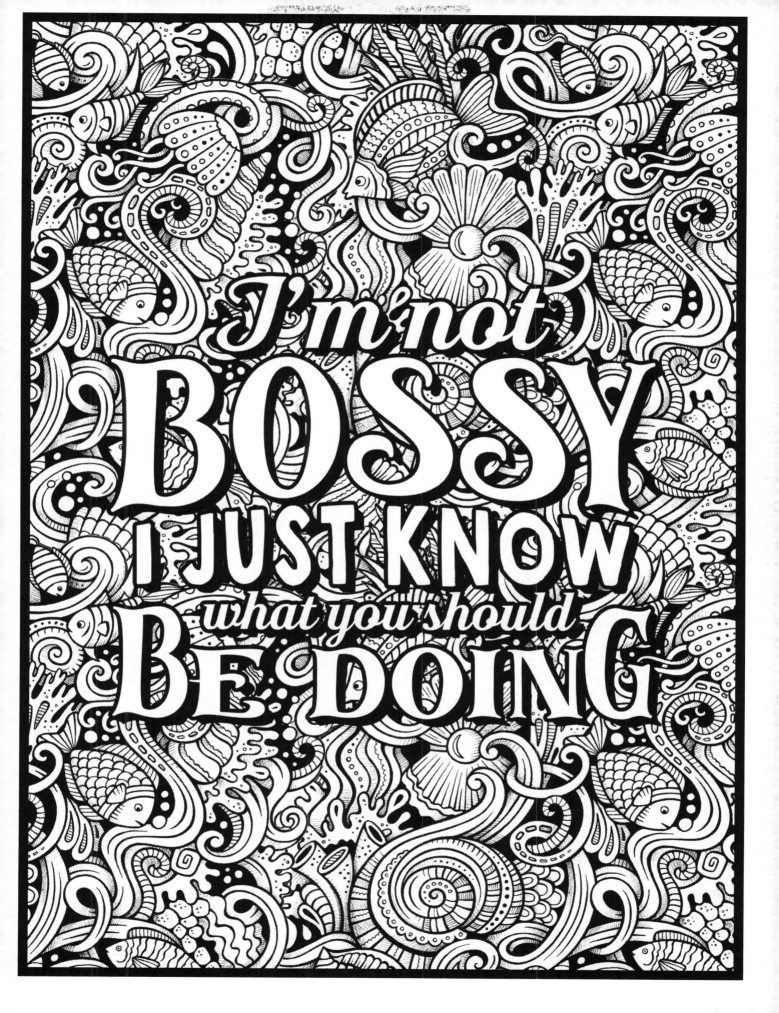

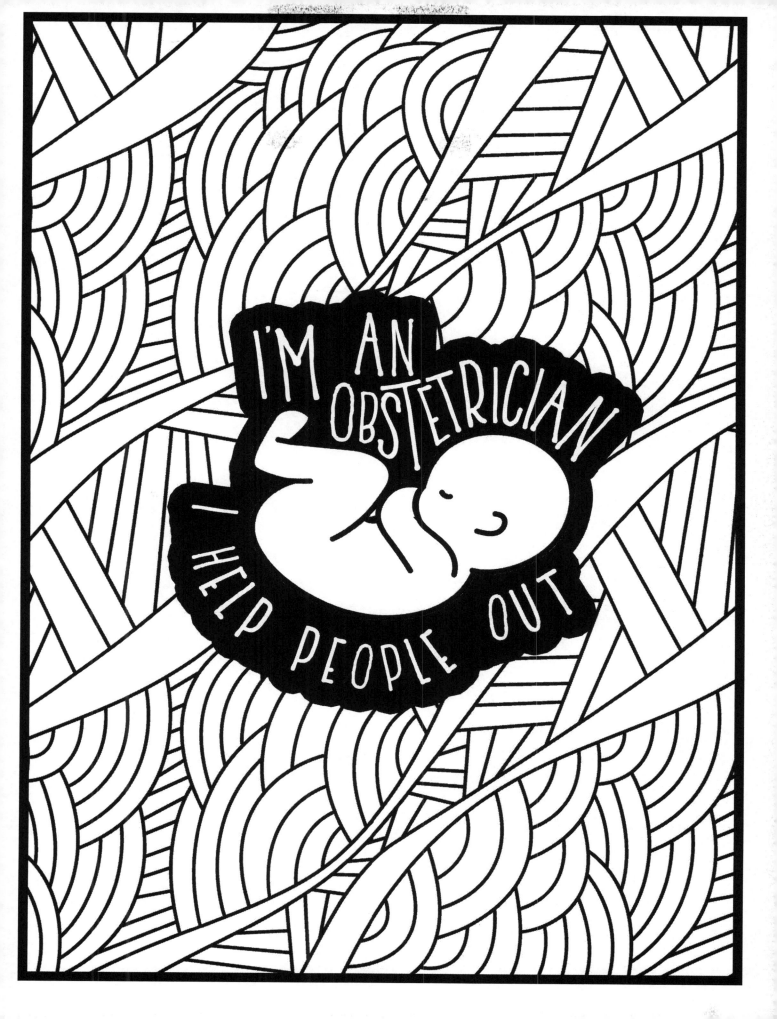

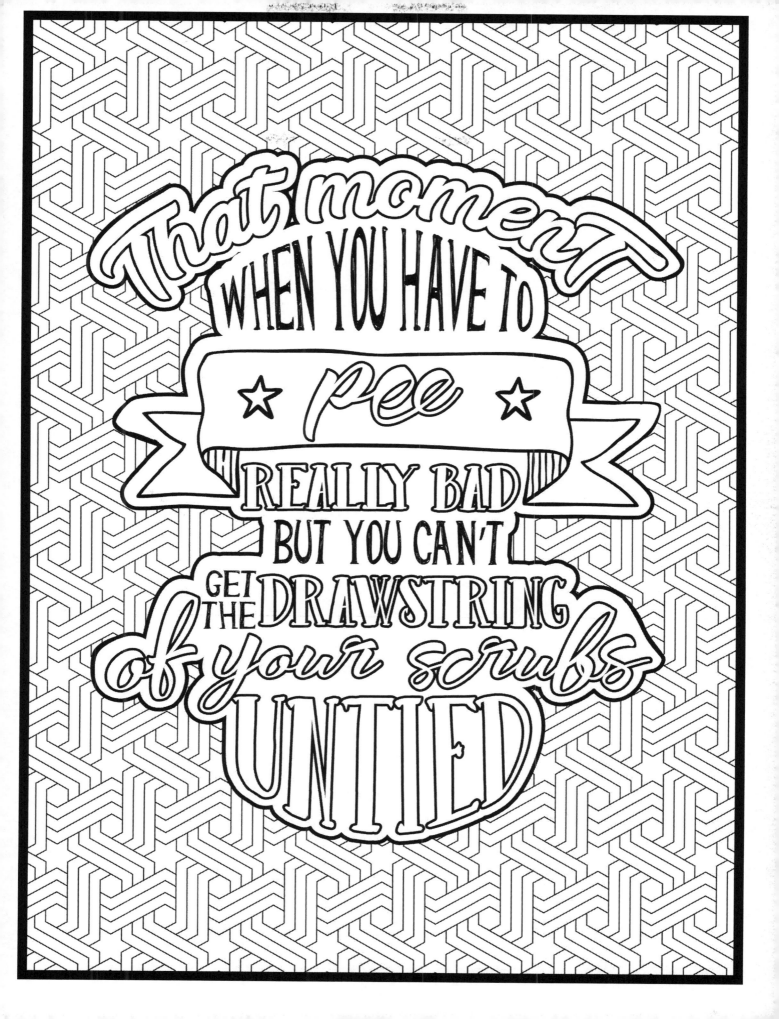

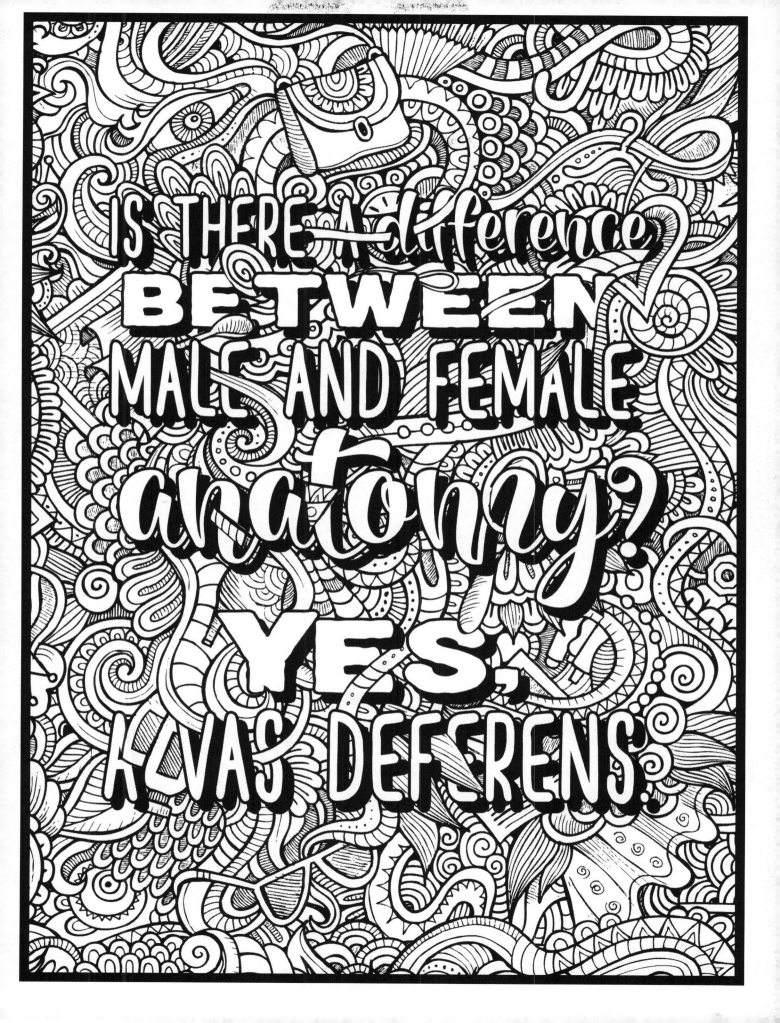

FREE PDF DOWNLOAD
OF THIS BOOK

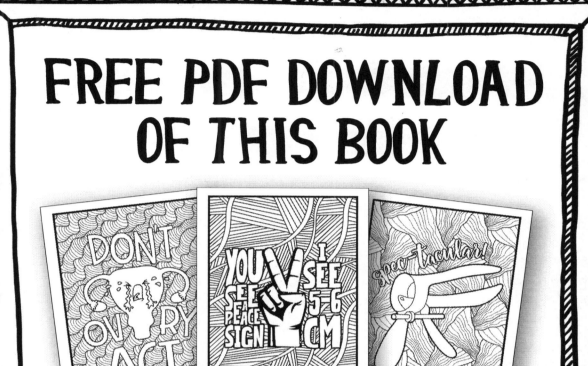

www.pbleu.com/baby

YOUR DOWNLOAD CODE: GYN373

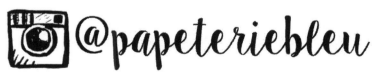 @papeteriebleu

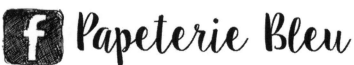 Papeterie Bleu

Want free goodies?
Email us at freebies@pbleu.com

@papeteriebleu

Papeterie Bleu

Shop our other books at
www.pbleu.com

Wholesale distribution through Ingram Content Group
www.ingramcontent.com/publishers/distribution/wholesale

For questions and customer service, email us at
support@pbleu.com

Made in the USA
San Bernardino,
CA

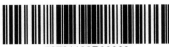

58731193R00060